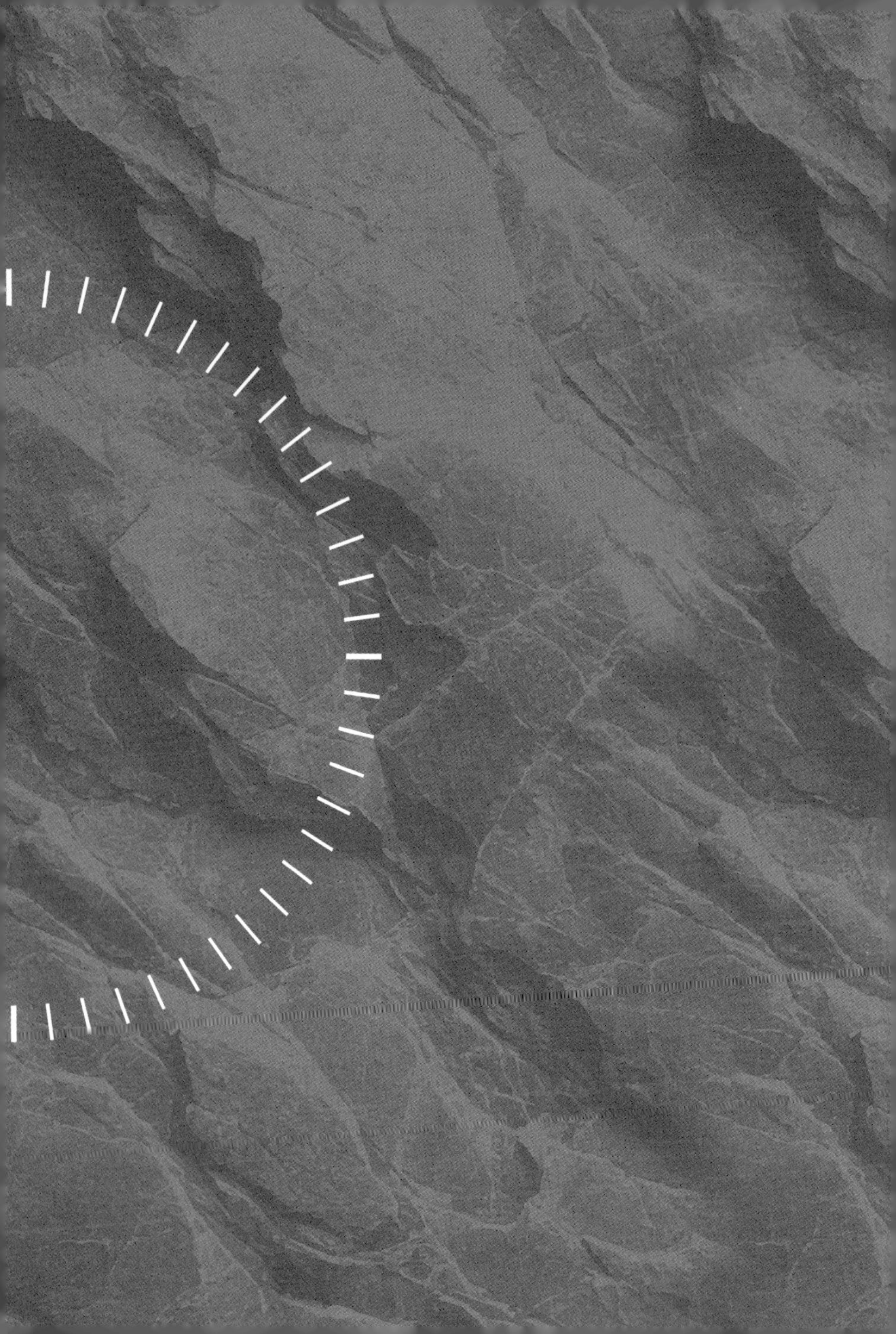

PRAISE FOR *THE NO-LIMITS LIFE*

Nordine has created what I wish everyone had within arm's reach: a powerful daily reset that's as grounded as it is energizing. The No-Limits Life blends hard-won wisdom with practical meditations you'll actually use—short reads that spark big shifts.

—**Bill O'Donnell**, Investor, Business Mogul,
and Founder of Miraval | *Life In Balance*

The No-Limits Life is a must-read for anyone wanting to enhance and boost the quality of their life. Everyone should seek it out.

—**Dharma Singh Khalsa**, MD, President and Medical
Director of Alzheimer's Research & Prevention Foundation

A powerful daily reset—clear, grounded, and deeply motivating. The No-Limits Life helps you build real strength, one choice at a time.

—**Jerry Avenaim**, Executive Director
of Mental Health Foundation

Nordine once again has provided us with the tools to become limitless. A must-read for all who want to improve their mind, spirit, and body.

—**VADM (ret.) Richard Carmona**, MD, MPH, FACS, 17th
Surgeon General of the Unites States of America,
and Laureate Professor at University of Arizona

If you've been stuck in your head, your fear, or your fatigue, this book brings you back to courage, clarity, and consistent action.

—**John Assaraf**

This is daily guidance for people who want more than motivation—they want transformation. It helps one keep promises, move promises to actions, and develop the discipline needed to make meaningful change in one's life.

—**Russell Redenbaugh**, Author of *Shift the Narrative: A Blind Man's Vision for Rewriting the Stories that Limit Us* and JJ Gold Medalist

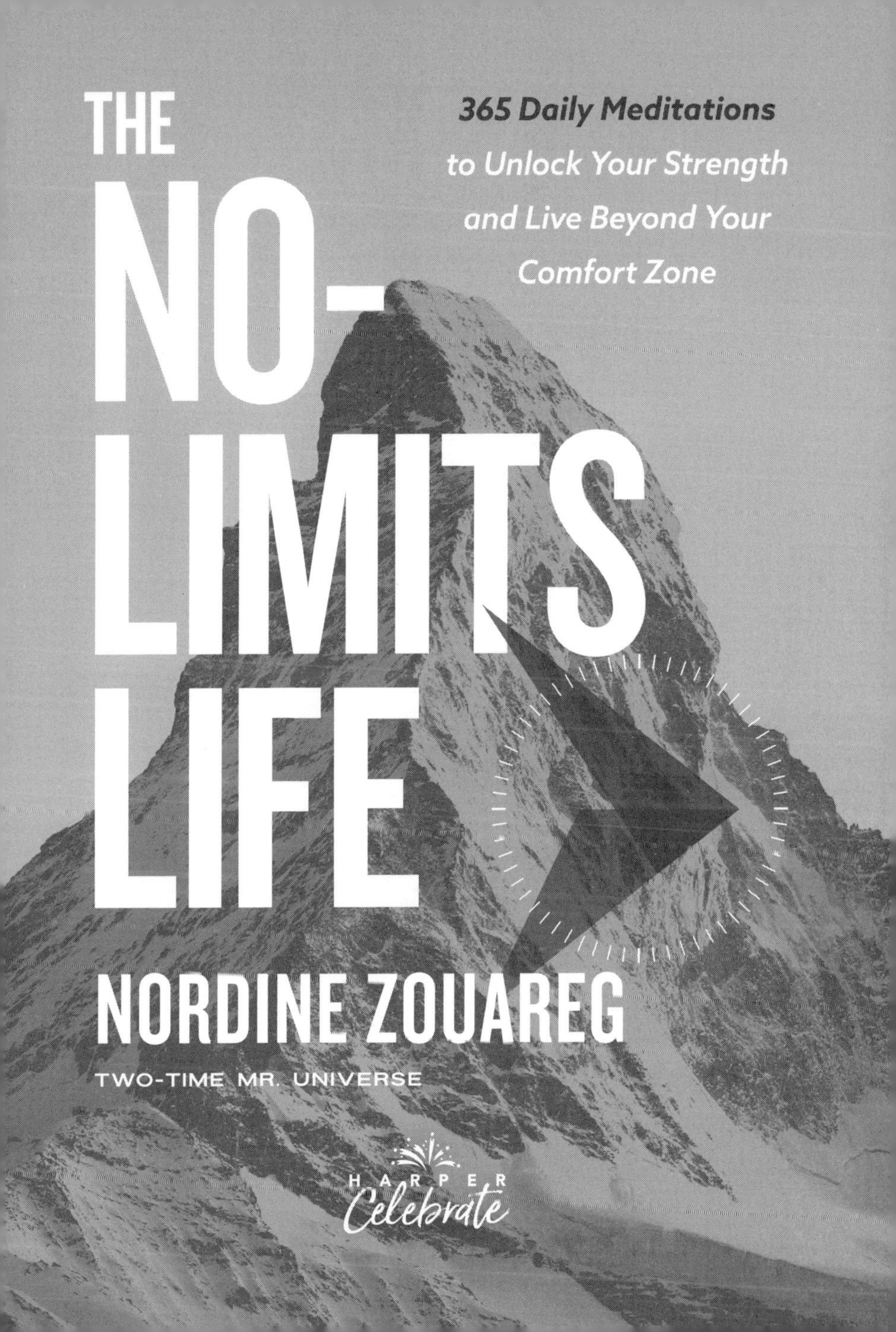

THE NO-LIMITS LIFE

365 Daily Meditations
to Unlock Your Strength and Live Beyond Your Comfort Zone

NORDINE ZOUAREG

TWO-TIME MR. UNIVERSE

HARPER Celebrate

For King, my companion, my healer, my mirror, who taught me that love without condition is the greatest strength of all.

The No-Limits Life

Published by Harper Celebrate, an imprint of HarperCollins Focus LLC.

Cover design and art direction: Sabryna Lugge
Interior design: Denise Froehlich
Author photo (back cover): VSL Creative

ISBN 978-1-4002-5575-7 (HC)
ISBN 978-1-4002-5577-1 (epub)

Printed in India

26 27 28 29 30 REP 5 4 3 2 1

CONTENTS

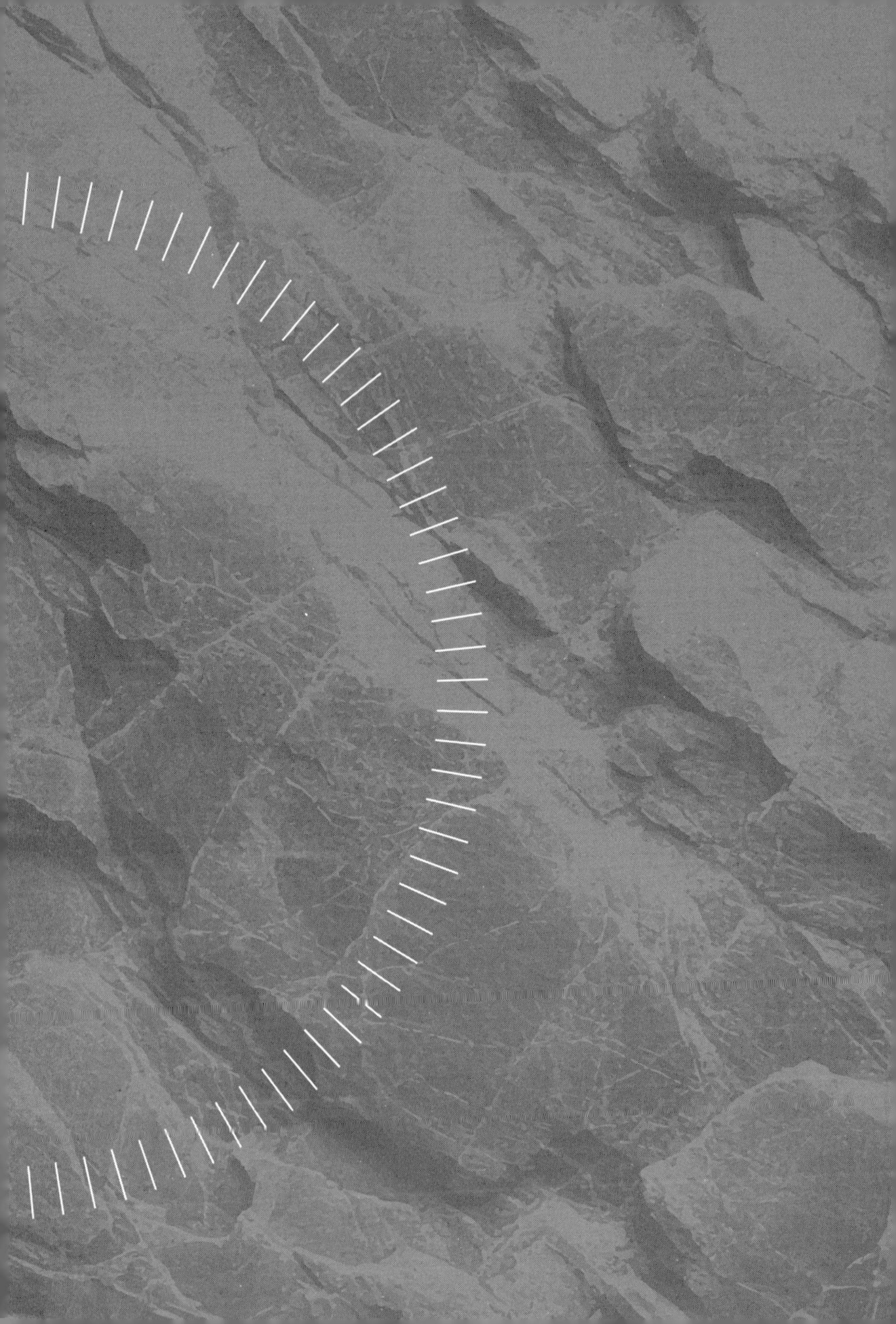

INTRODUCTION

The pages you're about to read aren't just words on paper—they are echoes. Echoes of grit. Echoes of pain. Echoes of triumph. They are the culmination of a lifetime spent chasing not just dreams but also the essence of what it means to live without limits.

These entries are a living chronicle of transformation—a mirror held up to the soul of a boy who dared to dream and became a man who refused to settle. These reflections are drawn from the trenches of life's fiercest battles and the summits of its most glorious victories. I wrote this book to remind you—and myself—that no matter how dark the night or distant the dream, there is always a path forward. A path carved by courage, paved by discipline, and lit by the fire that burns within each of us.

From Dreams to Reality: My Walk Among Giants

As a child, I had five heroes—Bruce Lee, Serge Nubret, Arnold Schwarzenegger, Sylvester Stallone, and Muhammad Ali—whose very existence whispered to me, "There's more to life than what you see."

My childhood heroes were larger than life. They were strength personified, resilience manifested, greatness in motion. While other kids were told to be realistic, I dared to believe that maybe—just maybe—I could one day stand where they stood.

Bruce Lee was the first. Though I never had the honor to meet him, his spirit ignited something deep within me. He wasn't just a martial artist; he was a philosopher, a disrupter, a force of nature. Bruce taught me that true power doesn't come from size or strength, but from alignment—of body, mind, and purpose.

Then there was Serge Nubret, nicknamed "the Black Panther" of bodybuilding. He was more than my idol—he became my mentor. I stood before him as a young, hungry athlete, and he saw something in me. Under his guidance, I learned that excellence isn't given. It's demanded—from within.

Arnold's path lit the way like a flare in the night. I didn't just admire it—I followed it. All the way to the stages where he had once stood. Mr. World, Mr. Universe. Titles that once seemed galaxies away were suddenly mine to hold. I honored his blueprint—and built my own legacy along the way.

Then came the moment I stood face-to-face with Rocky himself—Sylvester Stallone. The man whose on-screen journey awakened something primal in us all, a timeless truth that our deepest scars and our greatest victories are carved along the very same road.

And finally, the encounter that changed my life forever—meeting Muhammad Ali. To be in the presence of The Greatest, to hear his voice, to feel his energy, was a reminder that legends are real. And they aren't born. They're made.

With these heroes on my mind, every rep, every ounce of discipline, every sacrifice became a prayer to the altar of greatness.

Your heroes are guideposts, not finish lines. Let them inspire you, but never let them limit you. That's what *The No-Limits Life* is about. It's about breaking the illusion that greatness is reserved for the chosen few.

I wasn't born on the podium. I was born in the back of a military truck in the Sahara Desert during a sandstorm. The world tried to silence me before I had a voice. But my voice only grew louder. Stronger. And it carried me across continents and cultures and into arenas of both battle and beauty.

This Book Is for You

The No-Limits Life is a companion designed to walk beside you through your own journey, whether you're in the valley or on the mountaintop.

Each day, I'll guide you on your journey to live life with no limits. Every entry begins with a quote to spark inspiration and reflection. The personal story or lesson that follows connects the idea to real life, making it relatable and actionable. The takeaway distills the day's insight into a clear principle you can carry with you, while the closing question helps you pause, reflect, and apply the wisdom in a way that's personal to you. Together, these elements are designed to inspire both thought and action, helping you not just read but truly *live* each meditation.

You won't just be inspired—you'll be moved to act. To challenge the lies you've believed about yourself. To reclaim your voice. To rewire your mind-set. To remember that setbacks don't define you—your response to them does.

This book isn't about me. It's about *you*. It's about the champion within you that's been waiting for permission to rise. You won't find recycled motivation here. You'll find *real* lessons. Real scars. Real strategies. Because life isn't just about surviving hardship—it's about transforming yourself through it.

This is your invitation to step into your own arena and fight for the life that's already waiting for you.

From Surviving to Thriving

Make no mistake—this book wasn't born from comfort. It was forged in fire: in the pain of war, in the sting of racism, in the silence of betrayal, and in the noise of the inner critic. I've lived under the weight of colonization. I've tasted poverty. I've stood on the edge of mortality due to illness. I've weathered divorce. I've known what it feels like to build a life in a foreign land, starting with nothing but a name and a dream. I've faced financial ruin and watched opportunities slip through my fingers.

Yet I stand before you, not as a victim of circumstance, but as a testament to what's possible when the human spirit chooses to rise.

I share my life not to impress you, but to show you what's possible when you refuse to let life limit you. Pain is a brutal teacher, but a wise one. And the lessons it taught me—about character, courage, and clarity—are the very lessons I now offer to you.

It is the culmination of decades spent learning, breaking,

building, rising, and reaching again. It's shaped by the stage lights of global bodybuilding competitions, the spotlight of celebrity circles, and the quiet, sacred spaces of healing and coaching. I've shared rooms with billionaires and spiritual seekers. I've spoken with presidents and washed dishes in silence. Through it all, I've come to understand one thing: True success is not external. It's internal. It begins with knowing who you are—and who you refuse to stop becoming.

No Limits, Only Lessons

This book holds the echoes of giants. Lee, Nubret, Schwarzeneggar, Stallone, and Ali aren't just names to me. They are voices. Teachers. Catalysts. And their influence lives in every word I write. But make no mistake: *Their* legacy is not the point—and neither is mine. *Yours* is.

You have within you the same spark that lit their paths and mine. You don't need permission to be great. You don't need someone to hand you the script. You only need one thing: the courage to believe you already hold the pen.

Your story is waiting. Not in some distant tomorrow. But here. Now. In these pages. In this moment.

So turn the page. Begin again. And this time, let's do it without limits.

Nordine Zouareg

THE OTHER SIDE OF GREATNESS:

Coping with Anxiety

> The same mind that builds empires can also build prisons. Master the mind—and you master your freedom.

I've worn the crown of Mr. Universe. I've stood in front of packed rooms, trained Hollywood elites, coached CEOs, and changed lives. But behind the accolades, behind the muscles, behind the name, there's a boy who once shook with fear.

That boy was me.

Bullied, belittled, and bruised by the weight of racism while I was growing up in France, I carried anxiety before I even had a word for it. I didn't know what it was—I just knew I couldn't breathe. My chest would tighten, my thoughts would race, and no matter how much I accomplished, something inside me still felt unsettled.

Over time, I discovered something powerful: The same part of the brain that creates anxiety also creates greatness. The creative force that drives the artist to paint, the leader to build, and the athlete to dominate is the same fire that, left unchecked, can consume us from within.

High-performing people—yes, even your favorite entertainers and top-level professionals—often struggle with anxiety. Not because they're weak. But because they're intense. Passionate. Wired to push boundaries. And that energy, if not managed, can easily turn inward.

The good news? Anxiety doesn't have to control you. It can be understood. It can be worked with. It can even be transformed into fuel. In my journey, I've discovered ten powerful ways to cope with anxiety—tools I've used in my own life, and ones I continue to share with my clients around the world.

1. **Acknowledge it—don't deny it.** Denial delays healing. Naming your anxiety is the first step toward defusing it. You can't heal what you pretend doesn't exist. Courage starts with honesty.
2. **Move daily—let the body lead.** Anxiety is energy stuck in motion. Let it move. Whether it's a walk, a workout, or a stretch session, movement helps burn stress hormones and restore balance. The body knows how to process what the mind can't.
3. **Breathe with purpose.** Breath is life's rhythm. When anxiety spikes, your breath shortens. Flip the script: Slow down your breath, and you'll calm your nervous system. Try box breathing—inhale for four seconds, hold for four seconds, exhale four, hold four. Do this for five rounds.
4. **Fuel peace with nutrition.** What you eat affects how you feel. Minimize sugar, processed foods, and stimulants. Embrace whole foods rich in magnesium, B vitamins, and omega-3s. Your brain is an organ. It needs fuel, not fire.
5. **Sleep like you mean it.** Lack of sleep is like pouring gasoline on anxiety. Aim for seven to nine hours of uninterrupted, high-quality sleep. Turn off the screens, turn down the lights, and let your nervous system reset.

6. **Limit input—maximize presence.** Consuming too much media creates chaos in the mind. Set digital boundaries. Spend more time looking inward and less time scrolling outward.
7. **Practice mindfulness or meditation.** You don't need to levitate—just sit, breathe, and observe. Even ten minutes of mindfulness a day can lower anxiety and increase clarity. The present moment is where peace lives.
8. **Talk it out—don't just tough it out.** Silence feeds shame. Talk to someone—a friend, a therapist, a coach. Speaking out loud shifts the pressure. You were never meant to carry this alone.
9. **Journal the noise.** The mind is loud; the page is patient. Writing down your thoughts helps you separate what's real from what's imagined. Don't edit. Don't judge. Just write.
10. **Seek help without shame.** Getting support is not a weakness. It's intelligence. Strength isn't pretending to have it all together—it's knowing when to reach out. I've been there. And I promise, there's nothing weak about healing.

Anxiety isn't your enemy. It's a message. It's energy misdirected. But once you learn to listen, to respond, to care for yourself, you begin to reclaim your power.

I've lived the highs of fame and the lows of fear. And I'm here to tell you this: You're not broken. You're not alone. And you're more powerful than your anxiety.

You've got this—and I've got you.

JANUARY

IT STARTS IN THE MIND

Every transformation begins with a single, powerful thought.

Each new beginning or step forward begins in the mind—an idea, a spark, a quiet moment when something inside you says: *I can't stay the same. Something has to change*. And that's where transformation begins—not with action but with intention.

Before your body gets stronger, before the business expands, before your healing begins, a thought breaks through your doubts and you dare for a moment to believe something more is possible. That thought becomes the seed of change. You don't need all the answers. You don't need the perfect plan. You just need that one clear, committed belief: *Change is possible.*

Whether you're rising from defeat, rebuilding after loss, or simply choosing to evolve and grow, the first step always begins in the unseen space of your mind. Don't underestimate the thought that won't leave you alone, the idea that keeps jumping to the front of your mind. It might be your soul's way of telling you it's time for change.

Name that persistent thought that keeps bubbling to the surface. Let it guide your choices and fuel your momentum. You're only one belief away from becoming who you're meant to be.

What might happen if you finally let your thoughts lead the way?

DEFINE YOUR DIRECTION

If you don't know where you're going, you'll never get there.

Clarity is power. Without it, we tend to drift. We react rather than act. We stay busy but aren't fulfilled. We follow instead of lead. If you don't clearly define your direction, the world will define it for you—and it will rarely align with your true calling. Goals aren't just checkboxes. They're compasses pointing us in the direction we've defined for ourselves. When you know where you're going, your energy focuses, your time becomes purposeful, and your actions gain meaning.

If you're unclear on your destination, even small distractions can feel overwhelming and steer you off course. You may begin to question your worth—not because you lack ability but because you lack direction. The good news is you don't need to see the entire path to start. But you do need a destination. Even a single, specific intention can anchor you when life feels chaotic. Progress comes when effort is aligned with purpose.

Take time today to define your direction. Set one clear goal and map out the next few steps. Revisit this goal often, refining it as you move down the path. Success comes from choosing your path and walking it with intention.

What destination will you commit to defining today?

TAKE THE FIRST STEP

Don't waste time fearing what could go wrong. Just take the first step.

The beginning of any new journey is always the hardest part, not because it's complicated but because it's *uncertain*. We imagine all the ways it might fail, hesitating, revising, overthinking, and stalling. But clarity doesn't come *before* action; it's born *from* it.

You don't need to see the full map before taking that first step. Starting tends to bring the path into view, much like shining a flashlight reveals only the first few feet in front of you until you take one step forward, and then the next and the next.

Every great transformation, every bold reinvention, begins with a moment of *imperfect courage*. Fear will always whisper, "Wait!" But waiting rarely brings peace and often prolongs discomfort. Action, on the other hand, invites momentum. And momentum invites confidence. The real danger isn't in making mistakes—it's in never moving at all. Fear feeds on hesitation and starves in motion. Progress doesn't require perfection, only participation and the courage to keep going.

Don't wait for fear to disappear before chasing your dream. Move with the fear, through the fear, and toward what matters. Readiness is a result, not a requirement—so start before you're ready.

What one bold step could you take today if you stopped waiting for the perfect moment?

THE SHAPE OF DISCIPLINE

Discipline doesn't just shape your body. It builds the person you're becoming.

We often think of discipline as a harsh practice rooted in restriction or punishment. But with time and reflection, you may come to see it differently. Discipline is less about rigidity and more about alignment. It's the steady force behind real and lasting transformation—not just for surviving, but for evolving.

Yes, discipline in diet and exercise can shape the body. But that same discipline also shapes the mind. It clarifies our values, strengthens our character, and builds our self-trust. Every time we show up—whether for a workout, a promise to ourselves, or a choice that supports our well-being—we're casting a vote for the person we're becoming.

Discipline isn't about perfection. It's about consistency. And its power isn't in how loudly it shouts, but in how it quietly and steadily molds us—one decision, one action, one day at a time.

Reflect on your current habits. Do they support the version of yourself you aspire to become? Focus on consistency, not perfection. Choose one daily action that aligns with your goals—going on a ten-minute walk, eating mindfully, waking up on time. Every choice, no matter how big or small, is shaping you.

What will you build today—physically, mentally, and emotionally—with the tool of discipline?

PREPARE FOR THE CLIMB

No skilled climber takes on a mountain without both passion and preparation.

Pursuing big goals is a lot like climbing a mountain. Reaching the summit takes more than enthusiasm. Passion may get you started, but preparation keeps you going.

Many people set out toward a goal with fire in their hearts, believing that motivation alone is enough. But without a plan, without understanding the terrain ahead, without training and preparation, even the most passionate effort can end in burnout or discouragement. Purposeful climbers—those who reach the summit—don't rely only on adrenaline. They train. They anticipate setbacks. They study the route and pack the tools they'll need. And when they stumble, they don't give up—they adapt.

Whether your mountain is personal growth, a career change, or healing from past wounds, success comes from an approach that balances both vision and preparation. Sustainable progress, and ultimately reaching the mountaintop, happens when inspiration meets intentional planning and persistence.

Whatever mountain you're preparing to scale, ask yourself: *Am I equipped for this climb? Do my strategy and preparation match my passion?* Heart and desire may inspire you, but grounding and strategy will carry you to the top.

What tools, habits, or mind-sets can you put in place today so you can climb with purpose and confidence?

YOUR DREAMS AREN'T TOO BIG

The world is big enough for your biggest dreams.

Your dreams are not too much. They're not too big, too bold, or too late. The world is vast, and there is room for your voice, your vision, your purpose. Too often, we shrink ourselves to fit into the spaces we deem safe. We may fear there's already too much competition. Or perhaps too many others are already doing what we dream of. We live with a scarcity mind-set and believe that surely there isn't enough for all of us to succeed and flourish.

But the truth? No one else can do whatever your dream is quite like you. Your perspective is original. Your experiences are unmatched. And your presence, when rooted in courage and intention, makes room not just for you but for others too. The world doesn't need more silence. It needs your truth, spoken out loud. There is space here—for your story, your journey, your mark.

Stop waiting for permission to dream big. Step into your dream with boldness. Take one action today that affirms your right to be here, fully and unapologetically.

What might happen if you trust that there's room in the world for your dream?

THE HIDDEN TIDE WITHIN

Beneath a single emotion, many others are waiting to be felt—and to open the door to healing.

Emotions are layered. What appears to be irritation might be masking exhaustion. A moment of sadness could be carrying years of unspoken grief. And sometimes silence quietly hides a well of emotions stuffed tightly behind a locked door.

Many of us have been taught to push through, to stay composed, to be "strong." But real strength often reveals itself in vulnerability. The moment we allow ourselves to feel one true emotion, others follow. Beneath the surface, a tide of feelings is waiting for permission to surface. And when they do, they aren't there to destroy. They're there to reveal and to cleanse.

Giving ourselves space to feel these emotions isn't indulgent; it's necessary. Allowing ourselves to feel them doesn't mean giving up control. Instead, we're choosing to understand ourselves more fully. That single emotion you've been holding back might just be the gateway to clarity, release, and peace.

Create space today to feel an emotion you've been avoiding. Don't judge the emotion. Don't rush to fix or label it. Just notice what comes up and allow yourself to feel it. Emotional freedom starts with honest awareness.

Is there an emotion you're keeping hidden beneath the surface? What might shift if you allowed it to be felt?

THE CHOICE BETWEEN FEAR AND FAITH

Both fear and faith ask you to believe in something you can't see. It's your choice which one to follow.

Fear and faith are powerful forces, and both come into play when we're faced with uncertainty. In moments when we're forced to believe in something we can't see, whether we choose fear or faith determines where we'll go from there.

Fear keeps us frozen in the story of what might go wrong. Faith invites us to embrace the possibility of what could go right. Fear whispers doubts. Faith whispers courage. Fear pokes at your purpose. Faith inhabits it. Neither one guarantees an outcome, but only one moves us forward.

In the moments of uncertainty we'll inevitably face, we get to choose which voice to feed. You don't need to know what the path ahead looks like. You only need to believe, to take that first step toward faith. Because while the path of fear leads to hiding, the path of faith puts you on the road to becoming your full self.

The next time uncertainty arises, pause and ask yourself: *Am I feeding my fear, or am I nurturing my faith?* Choose to believe in your potential, even when the outcome isn't clear. Let faith guide your steps.

What part of your life is waiting for you to choose faith over fear? What might open up if you chose faith?

JANUARY 9

THE TRUTH BENEATH THE HABIT

True change comes when we stop fighting our habits and instead try to understand them.

We don't break habits by force. We may be able to will ourselves to stop an unwanted behavior for a time, but real healing comes when we transform those habits through understanding. The habits you struggle with most didn't show up by accident. They were born out of discomfort, fear, or a need for emotional safety. Then they became patterns.

True change begins with awareness. When you stop fighting and start listening, when you begin to ask what the habit is trying to protect you from, something inside will shift. You'll begin to move from shame to clarity, from control to compassion.

Parting with a habit isn't about erasing behavior. You're creating a new response to pain or need that is rooted in self-respect and love. This takes intention, consistency, patience, and, most of all, honesty. You can't heal what you won't face. But open eyes and an open heart can change everything.

> If you're trying to change a habit, don't ask how to break it. Ask *why the habit exists*. What story is it telling? What do you really need in place of what it is providing? Meet yourself—and those answers—with gentleness, not punishment.

What hidden truth is your habit disguising?
Are you ready to hear it?

THE WISDOM OF YES AND NO

Trust your yes. Honor your no.

There's quiet power in knowing when to say yes—and even more power in having the courage to say no. Your *yes* is sacred. It means you're all in, aligned, open. And your *no*? It's not rejection; it's protection. Your *no* draws the line where your peace lives, where your values stand tall, and where your energy remains whole and intact.

You don't have to explain your boundaries to everyone. You just need to respect them yourself. Because every time you trust your *yes* and honor your *no*, you're teaching the world how to treat you—and reminding yourself that your voice is worth listening to. This journey you're on isn't about pleasing others. It's about becoming someone you can be proud of.

And in case no one has told you lately, you're doing a great job. Keep going. Your alignment is your strength, and your honesty is your guide.

The next time you're faced with a choice, pause and ask yourself: *Is this an aligned* yes *or a peace-protecting* no*?*

Where in your life do you need to trust yourself more? What might change if you did?

JANUARY 11

THE SILENT THIEF

Self-doubt is the silent thief of abundance—it keeps you small in a world that's ready for your greatness.

Self-doubt rarely shouts. It whispers—quietly, constantly, on a loop. Self-doubt makes you second-guess your strengths, question your worth, and shrink in spaces where you were meant to rise. And the greatest danger of all is that self-doubt is *convincing*.

Self-doubt wears masks of humility, caution, logic. But underneath, it's fear disguised as reason. The cost? Dreams deferred. Talents buried. Opportunities missed before you even tried. Self-doubt convinces you to wait for permission that is already yours. The world doesn't benefit from you playing small. Your gifts, your vision, and your voice are needed. You weren't built to shrink so others will be more comfortable. You were built to grow, to stretch, and to step fully into the space that only *you* can fill.

Abundance isn't out of reach. It's waiting for you on the other side of belief.

Every time self-doubt shows up today, challenge it. You've earned your place in the world. You are not too much. In fact, you're *just getting started*. Let go of the lies that keep you small, and rise into the truth of who you are.

What part of your life is ready to grow—if only you would stop doubting it?

MOVE THROUGH IT

When the body finds rhythm, the mind finds calm.

Anxiety rarely responds to logic. You can't always think your way out of it because overthinking is often how it starts. Sometimes the most effective solution isn't mental—it's physical. One of the simplest ways to break anxiety's grip is by *moving* through the tension.

An anxious mind tends to loop, replaying fears and what-ifs. But your body can interrupt that loop. Movement grounds you. A simple walk, a light jog, even pacing the room—it shifts your chemistry. Moving your body reminds your nervous system that you're not stuck. That you have power, and rhythm is possible.

When your body finds motion, your mind finds permission to slow down. You don't have to move the fastest or the farthest you simply have to move with intention. Inhale. Exhale. Step forward. Let your body lead you to a place of peace.

When anxiety builds, don't freeze inside your thoughts—move with purpose. Let your body carry you back to calm. The way out is sometimes a single step forward.

What's one form of movement you can return to today, not to escape anxiety, but to gently walk through it, one breath at a time?

CHOOSING LOVE

Love doesn't survive on chemistry alone. Love endures through intentional connection.

While falling in love can feel like magic, staying in love is an act of will. That initial spark, the butterflies, the passion, the vision of a grand future may be effortless, but the flame that keeps love alive needs tending and demands consistency. Love isn't just something we feel; it's something we choose.

What sustains a relationship over time goes beyond passion and requires *presence*—giving quiet support when the other is struggling, forgiving when it would be easier to hold a grudge or turn away, showing up even when life gets complicated. Real love grows not in grand moments but in the small daily acts of care, honesty, and effort. It's not about never wavering—it's about choosing, again and again, to stay connected and committed.

Take a moment to reflect on how you're showing up for the love you've chosen. What small act can you offer today that speaks louder than words? A gesture, a kind word, your presence. Love that lasts is the love we choose, day after day, especially in the moments when it would be easier not to.

Are you choosing love today or just expecting it to stay?

AUTHORITY OVER YOUR MIND

Awareness gives you the power to choose what gets into your mind—and what doesn't.

We are constantly bombarded by media. Ads tell us who to be. Endless social media feeds inundate our minds with content. Talking heads attempt to shape how we think. Curated images influence how we perceive ourselves and others. Left unchecked, this constant stream can quietly erode our confidence and distort our self-worth.

But with conscious awareness, we can reclaim authority over our own minds. By observing and noting what we consume—both intentionally and passively—we can carefully consider its impact on our mood, mind-set, and motivation. Is your scrolling making you feel like your life isn't as good as everyone else's? Is the 24/7 newsfeed leaving your mind racing? Are you losing hours of your day to mindless consumption?

Awareness is your protection. By being mindful of what you allow into your mental space, you protect your peace, sharpen your focus, and deepen your connection with your true self and with the people around you.

Take a moment to become more aware of your digital diet. What are you feeding your mind? Are your daily inputs nourishing or draining you? Set boundaries. Unfollow what disturbs your peace. Lean into content that uplifts, educates, and inspires.

What can you filter out today to protect your inner clarity and focus?

LEADING THE MIND

The goal isn't to fight your mind. The goal is to lead it.

Many of us think that the only way to quiet the mind is by force. We must shut down negative thoughts, resist worry, push anxiety aside. But often, the harder we fight or resist these thoughts, the louder they get. It's like trying to silence a storm by yelling at the wind.

Peace doesn't come from controlling your thoughts. Peace comes from conscious leadership of them. You aren't in a battle with your mind. You are in a relationship with your thoughts, and you can guide them rather than try to control them. When you interact with your thoughts with the patience of a wise leader—curious, calm, and clear—you begin to influence them. Instead of wrestling with every fear or distraction, observe. Acknowledge and then gently redirect your focus toward what truly matters.

Leading the mind isn't about overpowering it—it's about choosing presence over panic, clarity over noise.

Next time your mind feels restless or overwhelmed, don't go to war with it. Take a breath. Note how you're feeling. Then guide your thoughts toward clarity, purpose, and truth.

Where will you guide your thoughts today—toward fear or toward freedom?

FROM TRYING TO DOING

Trying is subconsciously allowing yourself to fail.

There's a quiet loophole in the word *try*. It sounds noble. Effortful. Safe. But hidden beneath the word is often silent permission to back out.

Trying keeps one foot in and one foot out—committed enough to feel busy but not invested enough to be transformed. Saying "I'll try" cushions us from failure, but it also shields us from real success. Because *try* implies doubt. It prenegotiates the possibility of falling short.

But when you *decide*—when you *commit*—you step into a new identity. One that doesn't ask, *Can I?* but instead declares, *I will.* Trying might feel safer, but it's not where growth lives. Growth happens in *doing*, in *failing forward*, in showing up even when it's hard and even though you might fail. Growth happens when you stop seeking escape routes and start walking forward without looking back.

There's freedom in letting go of the word *try*. It's the difference between motion and progress. What if instead of trying, you just *did*?

Today, replace *I'll try* with *I will.* Speak it. Act on it. Notice how your mind and body respond to certainty over softness.

What goal have you been "trying" to reach when, deep down, you know it's time to commit fully?

CLOSED DOORS, CLEAR PATHS

Some doors stay closed to you because they're not meant for your journey.

It's natural to feel disappointment when a door doesn't open—when opportunity slips through your fingers, exciting plans shift elsewhere, or someone says no to something that really mattered to you. In those moments, it's easy to question your worth or direction.

But a closed door isn't always a rejection. Often it's redirection, a hidden form of grace. Sometimes we knock on doors that don't lead anywhere because we think they should. We chase validation instead of personal alignment. But true growth lives in spaces where we *fit*, not where we have to force our way in.

The opportunities meant for you won't require you to push. They'll open because you're ready. Because they match your path. And when one door closes, it often clears space for something better—something truer to who you're becoming.

Today, release the pressure to force what isn't flowing. Ask yourself: *Was that door about purpose—or approval?* Then breathe. Recenter. Redirect. The more you trust what doesn't open, the more prepared you'll be to walk through what does.

Can you think of a time when a closed door actually protected or redirected you toward something better? What did it teach you?

MORE THAN A ROLE

Your job is just one part of who you are. Don't let it consume you.

It's easy to get lost in roles, titles, responsibilities, achievements. Our careers can feel like the axis on which everything else spins. But a job—no matter how noble or demanding—is just one thread in the fabric of who you are. When work begins to define your identity, burnout will follow close behind. You become a title instead of a person. You forget the artist, the parent, the friend, the dreamer who still lives beyond those deadlines.

Your worth isn't measured by output. You are not your productivity. You are a whole human being—with feelings, needs, desires, and gifts that extend far beyond what is listed on a résumé or a performance evaluation. A fulfilling life doesn't sacrifice self for status—it balances both being and doing.

Take a step back today and ask: *What parts of me have I neglected in pursuit of performance?* Reclaim a passion. Call a loved one. Take a walk just for yourself. You are not your job. You are your *wholeness*.

What would your life look like if your identity wasn't tied to what you do but instead to who you are?

THE NEXT STEP IS YOURS

A mentor may open a door, but you choose whether to walk through it.

The guidance of a mentor is invaluable, but ultimately the responsibility for the next step lies with you. A mentor can share a wealth of knowledge, offer direction, and challenge your limits, but transformation still requires *your* courage, *your* discipline, *your* action.

Mentorship is both a mirror and a map. A wise mentor may help reveal the path, but they aren't the one who does the work. They may offer you tools, but they can't make you use them. The real growth happens when you use what has been given to you. Every insight becomes an invitation. Will you rise to meet it? Or will you stay where it's comfortable?

If you haven't already, consider seeking out a mentor. The mentor-mentee relationship flourishes when you take ownership, act with intention, and become an example whom others will one day learn from.

When you seek out mentorship, honor the opportunity being given to you. Show up fully. Follow through. Reflect, refine, and apply. When you act on the tools you've been given, you stop just being a student and grow toward becoming a guide.

How can you honor the wisdom you've been given? What will you do with that wisdom today?

HONOR THE RHYTHM OF SLEEP

When both mind and body release their grip and finally surrender, sleep has the opportunity to greet us gently.

Sleep can feel like a battle we're trying to win. We've all been there, tossing, turning, watching the clock, trying to will ourselves to rest, mind racing, thoughts taking the lead. But often the harder we try to force it, the more distant sleep becomes.

True rest doesn't respond to force but rather to surrender. When we stop replaying yesterday and rehearsing tomorrow, the mind softens, and often the body follows. We invite rest not by pressuring ourselves but through presence, mindfulness, and release. Sleep is our chance to return to a balanced state. It's a quiet homecoming for both body and mind.

When we approach sleep with gentleness rather than frustration, we open the door for rest to become not something we chase but a gift we receive.

As you get ready for bed tonight, shift your approach. Instead of "trying" to fall asleep, create a restful space, an environment of ease and calm. Turn down the lights, slow your breathing, and release the grip of spinning thoughts. Allow your body to feel safe to rest, and your mind free to drift. Trust that sleep will come—not through effort, but through stillness.

How will you create the inner quiet that invites sleep in tonight?

JANUARY 21

YOU ARE THE LIST

You're not just a line on a to-do list. You are the list.

It's easy to become consumed by the endless to-do list—meetings, deadlines, errands, obligations. You start checking boxes, but somewhere in the process, you forget to check in with yourself. You become a supporting character in your own life, placing your needs last, convincing yourself that rest can wait and that self-care is optional.

But here's the truth: Nothing runs well when the one running it is burned out. The to-do list becomes pointless if the doer has hit a wall. You aren't just another task to squeeze in. You are the foundation that everything else rests on. When you prioritize your sleep, your breath, your movement, your peace, each day will move differently. You will gain clarity. You will reclaim presence. You will lead from strength rather than depletion.

And this shift doesn't just benefit you. It empowers everyone who depends on you.

Look at your to-do list. Now look in the mirror. Are you present, cared for, and able to greet what needs to be done? If not, start again. Your well-being isn't selfish; it's strategic. When you honor yourself first, everything else aligns more gracefully.

What would change if your own well-being led each day, not as an afterthought but as the main priority?

ECHOES OF THE PAST

The past holds power only if you let it.
Those whispers are just echoes.

Your past may still speak, but it doesn't dictate who you are. Old wounds, regrets, and missteps may echo through your present, but they're just that—echoes. They're not commands. They're not the truth. They're just remnants of where you've been.

You are not the mistakes you've made, the heartbreak you've endured, or the loss you've felt. You are what you do next. And every time you show up with awareness, compassion, and courage, you're rewriting the next part of your story.

The past may try to remind you of who you were, but it can't define who you're becoming. You don't need to silence the past completely; it has something to teach you. But you can stop letting it steer the ship. The past can inform, but it does not get to imprison you. It can teach, but don't let it trap. Your freedom lives between the echo and your response.

The next time the past whispers in your ear, ask yourself: *Is this memory guiding me or holding me back?* Today is a blank page. Let your voice—not the echo of the past—write the next chapter.

What part of your past are you still listening to?
What would change if you took the pen back?

THE STARTING POINT OF UNDERSTANDING

True understanding begins when we
choose empathy over assumption.

Assumptions are mental shortcuts—quick judgments we make to feel safe or certain. But they rarely lead us closer to truth. They're often built from fragments of our past—fears, biases, or stories we've told ourselves to make sense of the unknown. And while assumptions close doors, empathy opens them.

Empathy asks something more of us. It asks us to pause the narrative in our heads and make space for someone else's story. It invites us to listen without interruption, to stay curious instead of drawing conclusions, and to recognize that we don't have to *agree* to *understand*. True empathy doesn't erase boundaries—it honors them. It doesn't require perfection, just presence. And in that presence, understanding begins to bloom.

When we choose empathy over assumption, we move from reaction to connection. We stop labeling and start learning. We quit distancing and begin bridging the gap between hearts and minds.

The next time you feel the urge to assume, stop yourself and get curious instead. Ask. Be willing to listen without preparing a response. Empathy is a choice, and it's the starting point of every meaningful connection.

Whose story have you yet to fully hear? How can you open the door for that conversation?

THE COURAGE TO TRANSFORM

Transformation isn't just a change in direction—it's the courage to align your life with what truly matters.

Change can be impulsive—a reaction to pain, pressure, or discomfort. But transformation is deeper. It doesn't come from fleeing what no longer fits but through stepping boldly toward what aligns with your truth. Transformation asks you to pause and reflect—not just on where you are, but on who you are becoming. When you release what once defined you, even if it still feels familiar, you take the courageous first step toward a real and sustaining transformation.

True transformation isn't about speed or spectacle—it's about sincerity. To transform is to stage a quiet rebellion against the life lived by default and to make a conscious return to the life built with intention. When you choose transformation, you're not just changing your path—you're honoring your purpose.

Ask yourself: *What parts of my life feel out of sync with my values?* Make a list of what isn't serving you. But don't rush to fix everything. Start with one shift, however small, that moves you closer to alignment with your values. The moment you act on what's true, transformation will begin.

What truth are you ready to honor with action today?

THE FOUNDATION OF GIVING

You can't pour from an empty cup. Nurture yourself first—and then you can better nurture others.

Giving is a beautiful act of connection, but when we give without boundaries or balance, we can slowly be drained of the very energy that fuels it. Many people pour endlessly into others—family, friends, colleagues—while quietly neglecting their own needs. Over time, this self-neglect leads to exhaustion, resentment, and burnout. What we seem to forget is that sustainable giving comes from overflow, not depletion.

Tending to your own well-being—emotionally, mentally, and physically—is not an indulgence. It's how you strengthen the vessel from which you give. When you're well rested, nourished, and emotionally grounded, the energy you share becomes more powerful, intentional, and authentic.

Pause today and take stock of your self-care habits. Are you fueling your body, calming your mind, and honoring your limits? Giving your best to others begins with giving something to yourself first. Create time for rest, reflection, and renewal. Remember: The most generous version of you starts with a nourished you.

What can you give yourself today so you can better give to others tomorrow?

ANGER CAN BE A SIGNAL

Listen to your anger. It is trying to tell you something.

Doubt can cause us to hesitate. Frustration sometimes pushes us forward. But anger? Anger has the power to derail us completely.

Anger typically flares quickly, clouding our judgment and leading to words and actions we later regret. While doubt and frustration can sometimes be redirected into determination or deeper focus, anger often consumes without direction. It's an emotional wildfire—burning fast, hot, and wide. But anger itself isn't evil. It's a signal. And it's often rooted in something deeper—pain, exhaustion, fear, or unmet expectations. When we treat anger as a sign, we gain insight instead of causing injury.

Anger will still visit. But when you pause, breathe, and ask, *What am I really feeling?* you shift from reaction to reflection. Giving yourself more insight and control over your response creates space for your power—not your impulse—to lead.

When anger shows up, instead of suppressing it, try to understand it. Use anger as a compass pointing to something unresolved, and then channel that energy into clarity and action rather than destruction. You are always stronger than the storm inside you.

How can you turn your next wave of anger into a moment of growth and grounded strength?

SUCCESS DEMANDS MORE

Success doesn't bow to the bare minimum.
Success comes to those who give their all.

Success isn't a reward for showing up halfway. Success is the result of full presence, full effort, and full belief. It doesn't answer to convenience. It doesn't show up for mediocrity. Success responds to commitment—the kind that doesn't quit when things get hard, the kind that keeps going when no one's watching.

You can't coast your way to excellence. And why would you want to? The real magic happens in the extra mile—in the effort you give when no one's keeping score, in the early-morning trip to the gym when you're tired, in the bold step you take when fear says, "Play it safe." Success is born not in the comfort zone but in the stretch.

Success asks for your time, for your heart, for your focus, for your grit. Give it your all, and success will become your reward.

Where in your life are you just getting by? Decide today to give more—not for applause but because your future deserves your full effort.

If you truly believe that success requires your everything, how could you show up differently starting today?

THE RIGHT TIME IS NOW

The right time to do the right thing is always now.

Many of us wait—for clarity, for confidence, or even for a sign that we're ready. But perfect timing is an illusion, and waiting for the perfect moment only delays the impact of our courage. Life rarely hands us the ideal moment wrapped in certainty.

In truth, progress begins the moment we stop waiting. The most meaningful shifts don't happen when everything is lined up just right. They begin when we decide to *act anyway.* Courage doesn't emerge from flawless conditions; it is born in motion, regardless of conditions. And the longer we hesitate, the more distant our goals become—not because we're incapable, but because we're frozen by indecision.

Every breakthrough starts with one simple decision: to begin.

If something is calling to you—a step you need to take, a truth you need to speak, a change you've been avoiding—don't wait for the perfect moment. Start now, right where you are. Even small steps create momentum, and momentum will build your strength. Trust that action will lead to clarity and that your courage is growing with each step you take.

What have you been waiting to do that you could begin today?

YOUR OWN MAGIC

Among eight billion souls, there is only one you—unrepeatable, irreplaceable.

In a world filled with noise, trends, and comparisons, it's easy to forget your own magic. But pause and consider this: Out of eight billion people, no one else thinks like you, feels like you, or walks your exact path. That uniqueness is your greatest superpower.

The more you chase someone else's definition of success or worth, the further you will drift from your own. But the moment you embrace who you are—your voice, your vision, your story—you will reclaim a kind of freedom that comparison can never offer.

You weren't meant to fit in. You were meant to stand out, to walk to your own rhythm, and to bring something to this world that only *you* can offer. Your difference is your distinction. Your presence leaves a mark no one else can replicate.

Let go of the need to imitate anyone else. Step fully into the truth of who you are. You're not a replica. You're an original masterpiece.

What part of yourself have you been hiding? What might change if you finally let that part of you shine?

ROUTINES VERSUS RITUALS

Routines fill our schedules, but rituals fill our souls—one is done out of habit, the other out of intention.

Routines are necessary. They bring structure, order, and predictability to our lives, helping us navigate responsibilities and get things done. But when we move through them on autopilot, even the most productive day can feel empty. That's where rituals come in.

A ritual doesn't have to be elaborate—it's any moment you approach with intention and presence. A morning coffee enjoyed in silence, a deep breath before a meeting, a moment of reflection at the end of a busy day—these simple acts, when done mindfully, can anchor us. They remind us that life isn't just about getting through the day but about being present in it.

When we elevate a routine into a ritual, we create space for connection, purpose, and peace.

Today, take one routine and transform it into a ritual. Add meaning. Add mindfulness. Add presence. You'll be surprised how even the smallest shift—from doing to *being*—can nourish your day and deepen your experience of life.

What routine will you elevate today? How will you transform it into something that feeds your soul?

THE TRUE COST OF WELL-BEING

Well-being isn't free—it costs your time, your choices, and your commitment to yourself.

Well-being isn't free—but we don't pay for it with money. The cost of well-being is your time, your energy, your discipline, and your self-respect. Every decision you make—what you eat, how you move, who you spend time with—either contributes to your well-being or quietly withdraws from it.

The truth is, you're always paying a price, either for your health today or for your healing tomorrow. And what do you receive in return? Energy that lasts, clarity that sharpens, peace that anchors, and strength that endures. These are the real dividends of well-being—the kind of wealth no paycheck can buy.

You don't have to be perfect. You just have to be intentional. Well-being comes from showing up for yourself, again and again, like your future depends on it—because it does.

Ask yourself: *Am I investing in my well-being or borrowing against it?* Choose one simple act today that strengthens your foundation. A nourishing meal. A deep breath. A clear boundary. Small deposits compound over time. Your future self will thank you—not just for how it made you look or appear to others but for how it made you *feel.*

What will you deposit into your well-being today?

FEBRUARY

PUT OUT THE FIRE OF ANXIETY

If you know the source of the flames of anxiety, why let the fire keep burning?

Living with anxiety can feel like standing in front of a fire—consuming, powerful, and hard to escape. At first, we hope the flames will die down on their own. But the more we avoid addressing the fire, the more we unknowingly fuel it. Avoidance becomes the oxygen that keeps the flames of anxiety alive.

Looking closer at what you're feeling is the first step to fighting the fire: *What is this anxiety really about? What am I afraid of?* Naming the core fear gives us power and brings clarity. And taking one small action—one breath, one journal entry, one honest conversation—can tamp down the flames and bring peace to your heart and mind. The fire may not disappear overnight, but it will begin to shrink.

The goal isn't to silence every anxious thought; it's to stop letting those thoughts run the show.

When anxiety rises up inside you, instead of fleeing, get curious: *What's feeding this fire of anxiety in me?* Then take a conscious step to reduce the fuel. Speak to a trusted person. Move your body. Write down your truth. Peace begins with awareness and grows through action.

What can you do today to reclaim your calm and begin putting out the fire of anxiety?

THE COURAGE TO FACE THE TRUTH

The courage to face the truth will set you free.

We often glorify truth as the key to freedom. As the well-known saying attributed to Jesus goes, "The truth will set you free" (see John 8:32). But truth on its own does nothing. It just sits there, waiting to be noticed, acknowledged, acted upon. Truth doesn't unlock doors or loosen chains unless you're willing to *turn the key.*

And that key is *courage.*

We may avoid picking up the key because the truth doesn't always feel good. We may be afraid of what the truth will demand of us. It can challenge our identity, our patterns, our comfort. It can dismantle illusions we've leaned on for years.

But here's the paradox: What may feel like confrontation is actually liberation. Avoided truth becomes a silent weight. Owned truth lightens your load. The moment you stop running from truth and start facing it in its entirety, you begin to reclaim your power.

Take a deep breath. Then ask yourself: *What truth am I pretending I can't see?* Name it. Face it head-on. You don't need to wait for the right moment. The right moment is *now.* The freedom you're seeking is on the other side of courage.

Are you willing to walk through the door that truth has already opened?

BREAK FREE FROM FEAR

If frustration, doubt, and unhappiness are weighing you down, stop making excuses and don't let fear hold you back.

Fear rarely shouts. It whispers lies and quietly lingers, convincing you to wait a little longer, to play it safe, to stay where it's comfortable.

But beneath frustration, self-doubt, or even apathy, fear is often hiding in plain sight. It tries to tell you that the timing isn't right, that you're not ready, that success belongs to someone else. And the longer you listen to the lies, the heavier life feels. The truth? The world isn't holding you back. You've given fear permission to lead—and it has taken over. But once you name fear, once you see clearly what it is, its grip lessens.

You don't need to leap. You don't need all the answers. Just take one honest, intentional step. Your happiness isn't waiting on perfection. It's waiting on courage.

Identify the fear behind your hesitation: *What fear is holding me back? If I faced it head-on, what could I gain?* Then take one step—however small—toward freedom. You don't need to have it all figured out. You just need to move.

What fear has kept you stuck? What would life look like if you left that fear behind?

RETURN TO YOURSELF

Every conscious breath is a chance
to return to yourself.

We all have moments of feeling disconnected, like our minds are racing in every direction and dragging us along for the ride. Overwhelmed by stress, paralyzed by fear, or simply numb, we can feel like we've lost touch with ourselves.

In those moments, we don't need to push harder or try to fix everything. What we truly need is a pause—a chance to return to center. This doesn't mean shutting off every thought or emotion but rather coming back to the part of us that remains steady and grounded, that feels true peace, even when everything else is uncertain.

That return may not be instant, but every conscious breath is one step closer. The mind may wander, but presence never leaves. And every time you choose presence, you come home to yourself.

When you feel scattered or overwhelmed, stop and gently ask, *Where am I right now?* Close your eyes and breathe deeply. Come back to yourself. Let that quiet space be your anchor. The journey back to you isn't a detour; it's the path.

What would it look like to return to yourself today? Are you willing to try?

AGING WITH GRACE

Growing old is a privilege, not a burden.

It's easy to view aging through a lens of loss—what parts of you move more slowly, what is changing in your mind and body, what no longer looks or feels the same. But aging isn't a failure of youth; it's the unfolding of this beautiful gift of life. Every year you live is a privilege many are denied. Each wrinkle, scar, and gray hair is not just a sign of the passage of time; it's a representation of survival, experience, and growth.

Youth may be glorified in our culture, but growing older gives perspective and wisdom that only time can reveal. Through this lens, aging deepens your gratitude, sharpens your clarity, and expands your heart. The stories you've lived, the wisdom you've earned, the grace you've learned to carry—these are the gifts of aging. You've earned them, so wear them with pride.

Aging doesn't take away your worth—it reveals it.

Shift your perspective today. Celebrate the privilege of another day, another chapter. Speak kindly to your reflection. Move with reverence, not regret. Age with intention, and let each year add another layer to your story.

What would it feel like to view every birthday not as another year lost but as more of yourself being revealed?

JOY AFTER THE STORM

Joy blooms brighter after we've been through the storm.

Real joy—joy that is forged in hardship—isn't fragile. It doesn't come from a life untouched by struggle but from the resilience built through the struggle. The storms you've weathered, the heartbreaks you've carried, the moments you thought you wouldn't make it through—they've softened you and strengthened you. They've cleared space for deeper gratitude, sharper perspective, and a more grounded kind of joy.

Joy that comes on the other side of pain is different. It's earned. It doesn't depend on circumstances—it grows from wisdom, from knowing that you survived, that you've grown, and that light can return. And when the light returns, it shines more deeply—not just around you, but *through* you.

This joy remembers. It honors the past. It's not loud, but it is lasting. You don't have to pretend the storm never happened. In fact, it's because of the storm that your joy now has roots.

Let yourself feel joy without guilt. You've earned it. Let it rise—not despite what you've faced but because of it.

What beauty in your life today was born from something you once thought would break you?

ALL YOU REALLY NEED

All you really need is love. The rest is life's way of adding a little extra beauty.

Many of us spend years chasing success, recognition, and comfort, believing they'll bring lasting fulfillment. But over time, life reveals a deeper truth: Without love, even the brightest achievements can feel empty.

Real love, whether for people, purpose, or simply being alive, is what gives meaning to everything. It's the anchor in chaos, the warmth during struggle, the light that makes the ordinary extraordinary. When we lead with love—toward others, toward ourselves, and toward the life we're shaping—everything starts to align. Wins feel richer. Losses feel softer. Even silence feels sacred.

Nobody can be perfect in anything—and love is no exception. But as long as you show up for love, it will continue to be there for you. And when we give love freely, life reflects it back in the most beautiful ways.

Look at your life through the lens of love. Where is love flowing freely? Where is it missing or in need of nurturing? Let love be your starting point and your compass. Everything else—success, recognition, beauty—will follow, not as the goal but as the gift that love naturally brings.

What needs to shift in your life for love to become a priority instead of an afterthought?

THE GIFT OF SHARED LIFE

Life feels fuller when it's shared—joy grows, burdens feel lighter, and everything starts to mean a little more.

Life's most meaningful moments aren't defined by what we achieve or where we are. What we remember about those moments is who we shared them with. A simple meal, a quiet walk, or an honest conversation can hold immense power when presence and connection are at the center.

No matter how strong we are, carrying life alone makes everything heavier. When we're on our own, success feels less sweet and struggle feels more isolating. But with the right people beside us, burdens feel lighter and joy expands. We're wired for connection, not just to be supported but to support. In those shared spaces, life becomes richer, deeper, and more fully alive.

True connection reminds us that we're not alone—that our stories matter, our emotions are valid, and our presence makes a difference. Through each other, we're able to remember what it means to truly live.

Who in your life brings meaning to your moments? Reach out today—not just when things are hard, but also during the ordinary days—to celebrate, to connect, to tell them you love them, or simply to be together. Share something real, and let connection bring more depth to your life.

How can you deepen your connections today so your journey feels less alone and more alive?

THE COURAGE OF CURIOSITY

The moment you ask, *What happens if . . . ?* curiosity becomes courage—and the path to wisdom begins.

Changing your life doesn't require a grand gesture. Sometimes, a great change begins with a quiet question—a pause between fear and action where you lean in instead of backing away. *What happens if I try? If I speak? If I let go?*

Curiosity is often mistaken for hesitation. But in truth, it's one of the boldest forms of courage. It dares to challenge what you've always believed, what you've been told, and what you fear might happen next. You open the door to learning, growth, and transformation through your willingness to explore the unknown.

When you trade judgment for inquiry and rigidity for wonder, your world expands. You stop needing all the answers before you take the step. Wisdom begins not in the knowing, but in the brave act of *wanting* to know.

Ask a question you've been afraid to ask. Let curiosity lead you where fear once ruled—and see what new doors open when you replace hesitation with wonder. Sometimes, the answer you receive isn't just information—it's freedom.

What are you brave enough to wonder about today, and where might that wonder take you?

PAIN CAN BE YOUR TEACHER

Growth starts where comfort ends.

Comfort may feel safe, but growth demands more of us. In both physical training and in life, real progress begins the moment things get uncomfortable. That burning muscle, that mental resistance, that emotional edge—it's there to invite you to the next level. In the gym, it's the last few reps, the ones you want to skip, that build the most strength. In life, it's the tough decisions, the difficult conversations, and the moments you feel like quitting that shape your character.

Pain is not your enemy; it's your teacher. Discomfort is not a barrier; it's a bridge. Those who grow the most don't avoid the challenge but instead lean into it. The struggle doesn't mean something is wrong. The struggle might just mean something powerful is happening and a breakthrough is on the horizon.

Where in your life are you playing it safe? Where are you letting the struggle stop you? Choose to stretch yourself today. Go one more rep; speak one brave truth; take one bold step. Push through. Your next level of strength is already waiting.

What resistance are you willing to face today in order to grow?

THE STRENGTH OF WILL

Your will is strongest when it's guided by faith. Without faith, the path will feel uncertain.

Willpower is a force—it pushes, persists, and endures. But even the strongest will can waver in the absence of deeper belief. When you rely solely on your own power, the journey can feel exhausting and aimless. Faith, however, gives willpower wings. It's not just about spiritual belief. Faith is the unshakable trust that your actions have meaning, that your purpose matters, and that every step you take is part of something bigger.

Faith turns resistance into resilience. It reminds you that setbacks can actually be setups and that delays are not denials. Together, your will and faith create a foundation that keeps you moving—with effort as well as intention and grace.

You don't need all the answers to keep going. But you do need a *reason*. And when your will is rooted in faith—in yourself, in your purpose, in something greater—no challenge can truly stop you.

Reflect today on the source of your will. Is it grounded in fear or in faith? Choose to lead with belief rather than rely on brute strength. When you let your will be guided by vision, not by urgency alone, endurance becomes transformation.

Where is your will leading you—and what deeper belief is guiding it?

THE MOSAIC OF YOUR LIFE

We aren't meant to live just one life. We're called to live many lives within the same lifetime.

You aren't limited to one path, one identity, or one version of yourself. The journey of life isn't a straight line but rather a series of evolutions. It's easy to see that who you are today isn't who you were ten years ago, but sometimes you might forget that you're not stuck in the place you are today.

Who you're becoming may surprise you. Growth demands reinvention. You may be called to release roles you've outgrown—careers, relationships, mind-sets. Those prior paths weren't necessarily wrong. You've simply expanded beyond them.

Each version of you serves a purpose. Some phases teach you strength; others cultivate humility. Some ignite ambition; others soften you toward compassion. You are a mosaic of every chapter you've lived, every identity you've tried on, every truth you've dared to explore.

Don't fear the transformation. Instead, embrace the amazing truth that you're allowed to evolve.

Ask yourself: *Am I clinging to an outdated version of myself just to feel safe?* If you are, resolve to let go. Make space for the next version of you to rise—bolder, wiser, freer.

What part of yourself are you ready to outgrow so you can step into who you're meant to become next?

WHERE LOVE GROWS STRONGEST

True connection is built on freedom, not control.

The most meaningful relationships are built on mutual respect and emotional freedom, not control. If you've ever been in a relationship that caused you to fear or feel insecure, your instinct may have been to slip into control—checking on the other person, seeking constant reassurance, setting unspoken expectations, clinging to the belief that containment equals closeness. But control stifles connection, erodes trust, dims authenticity, and turns love into obligation.

The most rewarding relationships, the ones that truly nourish us, don't thrive in fear and control. Both people feel safe to be fully themselves. Individuality is honored, not feared. Giving space to grow isn't seen as distance but as depth.

When we give others the freedom to be who they are, love breathes easier. It expands. Instead of shrinking us, real love frees us, expands us, and supports us as we rise.

Reflect on the relationships in your life. Are they grounded in freedom or weighed down by control? Does fear cause you to grasp tightly rather than opening your heart to trust, communication, and respect? Love grows strongest when it isn't caged and is given room to breathe.

How can you create more freedom and trust in the way you connect with others?

THE SPACE BETWEEN

Lasting love is about honoring your individuality and growing stronger in the space between.

Connection isn't born out of sameness—similar likes and dislikes, similar goals, a desire for the same outcome. True connection is forged in the space between two whole people who choose to meet, again and again, with presence and respect. Real love between friends, family members, and partners doesn't demand that we be identical. Instead, we are invited to stand side by side, grounded in our own truths, while still reaching toward one another with open hands and open hearts.

When we try to mold someone into our mirror, we lose the richness that uniqueness brings. But when we honor our differences—distinct perspectives, contrasting strengths, quiet ways in which we stretch one another—we create a deeper intimacy.

The space between—filled with listening, learning, and loving—is where the real growth happens and where love endures.

Ask yourself: *Am I loving this person for who they are or for who I want them to be?* Be honest. Then let your love breathe and stretch. Honor the space between you and the other person.

What part of your relationship needs more room to grow, not by becoming the same but by choosing to honor your differences?

ACKNOWLEDGE YOUR WINS

A high-five to yourself is a quiet act of self-recognition—proof that you're still showing up, no matter what.

There are countless moments in life—whether in public achievements or in quiet personal battles—when no one is around to cheer for us. It's easy to believe that encouragement counts only when it comes from others. But some of the most meaningful validation comes from within.

A simple "I'm proud of you," whispered to yourself.

A smile in the mirror after pushing through something difficult.

A deep breath after holding your ground or showing up when it would have been easier to bail.

These moments matter. Inner recognition is powerful. It reminds us that we're still standing, still evolving, still choosing to show up. And sometimes, that quiet self-acknowledgment is enough to not only keep us going but also to give us the recognition we need.

Take a moment today to acknowledge a win. It doesn't have to be loud or public. Look in the mirror and say, "I'm proud of you." Celebrate the fact that you're still showing up—still doing the work, still choosing to grow. A high-five to yourself may seem like a small gesture, but it could unlock the strength you need to keep going.

When was the last time you gave yourself credit for staying the course? How did that feel?

WHEN TO SAY NOTHING

True wisdom lies not in how much you say
but in knowing when to say nothing.

In a world obsessed with instant responses and constant noise, silence is often misunderstood. Silence can be seen as weakness, but to the contrary, silence is presence without pressure. It's the space where clarity gathers and truth begins to rise.

You don't always have to respond. You don't have to fill the gap, to bridge the silence with your voice. The wisest voices are often the most quiet ones not because they lack something to say but because they know when their words will *truly* add value. Silence gives you time to feel, to process, to choose deliberately instead of reacting impulsively.

The next time you find yourself in a moment of tension, discomfort, or urgency, pause. Breathe. Take note of the space you'd normally rush to fill. That space is sacred. What you *don't* say in that moment often communicates more about your wisdom than anything you could rush to explain.

Resist the urge to fill every silence. Be mindful today before you speak. *Is what I'm thinking of saying necessary? Is it kind? Is it true?* Let your words carry intention, and let your silence carry weight. Wisdom doesn't always speak, but it always listens.

Where in your life could silence bring more understanding, presence, or peace?

FEBRUARY 17

THE SANCTUARY OF HOME

Make home your sanctuary—a space for rest, connection, and renewal.

The spaces we live in often reflect the state of our inner world. When our environment is calm, clean, and intentional, it supports and reflects a sense of peace and clarity. But when clutter, chaos, or constant distraction fills the space, that echo often reveals the stress we're carrying inside.

Our homes—whether large or small—should be more than just places we occupy. They should be sanctuaries. Spaces where we can breathe, reflect, and return to ourselves. Modern life moves fast and demands much of us, and having an environment that restores rather than depletes is essential.

Creating this kind of space doesn't require perfection. Instead, step into alignment by tending to what's around you. Your outer world and your inner world mirror one another, so when you make small, intentional changes in your environment, you invite calm within. As the two come into balance, harmony takes root, and that harmony becomes a sacred space for rest, resilience, and renewal.

Look around your space—does it bring you peace or tension? Clear one corner, open a window, light a candle. Protect your space, and it will restore you.

What one action can you tako today to make your home a haven?

THE POWER OF STILLNESS

When you become still enough to hear your own heartbeat, you're able to hear others' hearts speak.

Our lives are in a constant state of busyness and motion. Stillness can feel unnatural, uncomfortable even. But stillness isn't a pause on life before we get back to what matters. *Stillness* matters. It's a powerful part of our lives we need to pay attention to. It helps us to hear the quiet truths we often overlook. It allows insight to surface, emotions to clarify, and connection to deepen.

When we quiet the external distractions, we can finally tune in to what matters: our breath, our values, and the presence of others. You're not withdrawing from life; you're actually arriving in it more fully because you are present.

Stillness invites us to lead with presence, speak with intention, and connect with empathy. From that place, we not only hear ourselves more clearly—we become more attuned to the unspoken language of those around us.

Give yourself five minutes of quiet today. No phone, no distractions, just your presence. Listen to your breath, feel your heartbeat, and simply be. Let stillness expand your awareness—not just inward but outward toward others. When we're still enough to connect with ourselves, we're better able to connect with the world.

What might you discover if you gave yourself permission to be still more often?

FROM VISION TO REALITY

What the mind dares to envision with clarity and conviction, the hands will eventually shape into reality.

Everything begins in the mind. Every achievement, every breakthrough, every revolution first existed as a single thought. But thought alone isn't enough. Every thought needs clarity to focus it and conviction to fuel it and transform it into action. When you truly *see* your vision—when it lives in your mind not as a fantasy, but as a calling—your actions begin to align. Your hands follow your belief.

Clarity gives you direction. Conviction gives you endurance. Together, they build momentum, and momentum turns dreams into form. You don't need to have all the steps figured out. You just need to keep showing up with a mind that sees *what's possible* and a will that refuses to stop building toward it.

Your reality is not something you live in passively. When you have the courage to imagine something greater, you create your own reality.

> Do not dismiss your vision as "too big." Identify it. Strengthen your belief in it. Then let your hands begin the work of shaping it into the world.

What vision have you been holding yourself back from pursuing—and what's one action you can take today to bring it closer to life?

TRUST THE WAIT

Once the seeds are planted, the best thing you can do is trust the wait.

We live in a world that rewards speed—fast answers, instant results, quick fixes. But the most meaningful things in life don't bloom on demand. They grow in silence, in hidden places, in time. The seed you planted—whether a dream, a habit, a healing journey—needs time to take root before it peeks up through the surface. And while it may feel like nothing is happening, *everything* is happening beneath the surface.

Patience isn't about doing nothing. Patience is an active form of trust. It's saying, "I believe in the process even when I don't have proof." And that trust becomes the soil in which growth thrives. Rush the process, and you risk disturbing what's trying to take shape. Stay steady, stay present, and the harvest will come—stronger, fuller, and more abundant than anything you could have forced.

Honor the waiting. Water your vision with consistency, not control. Step back and trust that what you've planted will rise when it's ready.

What part of your life is quietly growing beneath the surface? Can you trust it enough to give it time?

FEBRUARY 21

ACCEPTING REALITY

"It is what it is . . ." But what exactly does that mean?

"It is what it is" can feel like a shrug, a trite way to bypass discomfort. But when we examine it more closely, we'll find it holds a deeper wisdom.

Acceptance isn't the same as giving up. When you choose to accept, you are able to let go of the battle with circumstances you can't change and can instead focus your energy where it counts. This approach isn't passivity; it's presence. When you accept something, you're not saying it's ideal. You're simply acknowledging reality, without distortion or denial. And from that grounded place, you can choose how to respond with clarity rather than resistance.

Acceptance frees you from the weight of "should haves" and "what-ifs" and plants you firmly in the now. Accepting doesn't mean you've decided to stop growing. You simply aren't going to waste precious energy fighting reality. And from that perspective, new wisdom will rise.

Practice saying, "It is what it is" with intention—not to dismiss whatever is going on but to center yourself. Notice where you're resisting what is already true. Can you surrender to reality and look for your next empowered step?

Where in your life are you mistaking resistance for strength when acceptance is inviting you to move forward?

THE QUIET VICTORIES

Don't count the tasks left undone—count the quiet victories, the steps no one sees.

It's so easy to focus on what is unfinished—the unchecked boxes, the goals still out of reach. But real progress rarely makes a loud entrance. True and lasting growth happens in the quiet moments, in those seasons of dedication when no one cheers you on or even notices—waking up early when you wanted to sleep in, choosing grace over frustration, taking a single step forward when it would have felt more comfortable to stay put.

These small victories don't make headlines, but they build resilience, discipline, and trust in yourself. The world may not notice, but your future will. Even the smallest wins plant seeds of momentum. Over time, those seeds become habits, and those habits ultimately shape your future.

Every quiet victory is a promise kept to the version of you that refuses to quit.

Shift your focus today. Instead of measuring what you haven't done, honor the unseen wins you've already achieved. They are the foundation for growth, the small wins that move you forward.

What quiet victory did you earn today? Have you paused yet to celebrate it?

THE SCULPTOR AND THE STONE

Accountability is about shaping yourself with honesty and courage.

Accountability can get a bad rap, especially if people don't understand it. It may sound like pressure, blame, or a constant checklist of things you should've done better. But real accountability is different: It's about strength, not shame. The moment you stop waiting for someone else to fix, rescue, or define you and start shaping your own growth, integrity, and peace, you step into the true power of accountability. To embrace accountability is to be both sculptor and stone. You're shaping who you become, one honest choice at a time. It takes courage to look in the mirror and say, *This part of me needs work*. But in that moment, you're not naming your weakness for all to see; you're embracing the freedom to course-correct, to rebuild, to grow.

Accountability doesn't translate to perfection. It asks only that you stay *in process*—with compassion, with clarity, and with a commitment to your higher self.

> Stand in your truth—not by trying to control everything but by claiming responsibility for what is yours to shape. Stop hiding and start carving. You're the artist of what you are becoming.

Where in your life are you waiting for change when you actually need to be taking ownership?

UNLOCKING INNOVATION

You don't need to reinvent the wheel. You just need to refine what's already working and make it your own.

In a world driven by disruption and novelty, we often overlook the quiet power of refinement. Our culture pressures us to always be doing something radically new, to chase the next big thing, to hop on the latest trend. But true innovation doesn't always come from reinvention. It comes from doing what already works—only better. Sometimes the smallest adjustments unlock the greatest progress: a shift in routine, a clearer system, a simplified process, a change in environment.

These subtle refinements often move us further than a sweeping change ever could.

Seeking innovation through a lens of simplicity isn't the absence of creativity. Rather, it's a sign of mastery. A simple, grounded approach reveals a deep understanding of what matters and eliminates what doesn't. When we stop overcomplicating and start optimizing, we tap into a more sustainable kind of growth—one that's rooted in clarity and intention.

What's already working in your life? How could it work even better? Zoom in. Refine your habits. Simplify your systems. Don't confuse motion with progress. Sometimes the smartest move is not to do more but to do whatever it is with *more purpose.*

What one area of your life are you ready to fine-tune for deeper, lasting impact?

BEYOND VICTORIES AND DEFEATS

True growth lies in knowing which actions shaped your path and which were simply missteps along the way.

You are not your wins. And you certainly aren't your losses. The scoreboard—whether in your favor or not—is no indicator of your worth. The way you rise up, recalibrate, and keep moving after a setback or a win is what defines your path.

There will be seasons when everything aligns and you feel unstoppable. At other times, it'll feel like nothing is going your way—defeat will humble you and doubt will creep in. But neither state is permanent, and each moment is an invitation to grow.

You don't need the world's applause to prove your progress. Your victory is found in the quiet discipline it takes to keep showing up, the courage to keep refining your mind-set, and the wisdom to learn from mistakes without letting them steal your momentum.

Don't cling to wins or crumble from losses. Instead, ask yourself: *What did I learn? What will I do differently the next time?* That's how you evolve. That's how you lead yourself forward—resilient, focused, and unshaken.

Which recent experience taught you more: your most recent success or your latest setback? How will you grow from it?

HOW FORGIVING FREES YOU

Forgiveness isn't only for the one who receives it. It's for the one who gives it too.

Forgiveness is often misunderstood. It's sometimes seen as a soft choice, even a sign of surrender. How is the offender held responsible if we forgive them? On the contrary, forgiveness is one of the strongest actions we can take—not only for whoever has harmed us but also for ourselves.

Your anger, resentment, or pain may be justified. And carrying it may feel protective. But over time, those emotions can become chains, weighing you down and holding you back, the pain lingering as you continue to carry it. Choosing to forgive doesn't mean you deny what happened or excuse the wrongdoing. It doesn't even mean you have to be involved with that person again. Forgiveness does mean reclaiming your peace, clarity, and freedom.

More than a gift for the person who hurt you, forgiveness is a gift you give yourself. Forgiveness allows you to step out of the past and into your future—whole, unburdened, and free.

Ask yourself: *Is holding on to this pain helping me grow or keeping me stuck?* Forgive and let go—not because the other person deserves it, but because *you* deserve it.

What emotional weight are you willing to lay down today so you can rise lighter and stronger tomorrow?

THE WISDOM OF HUMILITY

Don't let success go to your head.
Humility clears what pride clouds.

Many of us have experienced moments of success accompanied by praise, recognition, and validation. At first, it feels great—like confirmation that we're important, that we're "good," that we're enough. But when we let external praise shape our identity, we may sacrifice openness and growth.

Pride can be so subtle, so insidious. Pride whispers that we've arrived, that we're on top, that we no longer need input, when in truth, we're only just beginning. Pride also reveals the truth behind the phrase "how the mighty have fallen." The mountaintop can be precarious if we're not paying attention.

Humility is a grounding force that keeps us anchored. Humility doesn't ask that we dismiss our achievements but that we not be defined by them. No matter how much we accomplish, we are never done learning and growing. True success is found in how we quietly continue to evolve—before, during, and after the roar of applause.

Take a quiet moment today to look at your recent wins. Celebrate them, yes—but also ask yourself: *Am I staying open? Am I still learning?* Let humility keep your heart clear and your mind open.

How might humility help you succeed—while not losing sight of what matters most?

WHEN INTUITION MEETS CONFIRMATION

When someone's advice aligns with your gut feeling, take it as a green light.

You've felt it before—that quiet instinct, that voice whispering beneath the noise. It may not always be loud, but if you're listening, it's there. And when someone else's guidance echoes what you already sensed deep within, it's not coincidence—it's *confirmation*.

A moment like this isn't a sign that another person knows more than we do. When someone speaks into our lives in a way that resonates, our intuition is being validated—reflected back to us from another angle. It's the universe's way of reminding us that we can trust ourselves, and that truth often travels in harmony.

Too often, we second-guess our instincts, waiting for proof. But your gut is inherently attuned to truth. It speaks in nudges, in quiet knowing, in patterns only you can trace. When outside wisdom matches inner clarity, you can feel confident that you're aligned and ready to move forward. Trust that alignment.

Stop waiting for permission. If your heart and your intuition are speaking the same language and someone else is confirming it, consider the path open. Sometimes that second voice, backing up your inner knowing, is just the nudge needed to help you take the next step.

What quiet knowing have you been resisting? Who or what has echoed it?

FEBRUARY 29

THE POWER OF BOLD MOVES

Sometimes a quantum leap is the only way to break free from being stuck.

When you feel stuck, it's tempting to take small, safe steps, hoping that incremental progress will follow. But sometimes, those little steps only keep you orbiting the same problem.

In some moments, the only way forward is a bold leap—a decision so clear, so courageous, so extreme, that it disrupts your patterns and creates space for something new. Contrary to what you might believe, boldness isn't recklessness if it's grounded in trust—trust in your ability to adapt, to grow, and to figure it out as you go.

You don't need to have every answer. You just need to be brave enough to move when your soul says, "Go!" The most powerful breakthroughs often come from the scariest leaps.

If you've been circling the same question, the same fear, the same hesitation, maybe it's time: Leap. Say yes. Walk away. Start fresh. End it. Choose the move that shakes you awake. Boldness is the bridge to your next chapter.

Where in your life have you been tiptoeing when, deep down, you know it's time to leap?

MARCH

THE FORMULA FOR GREAT RELATIONSHIPS

Relationships become complicated when we forget their true purpose.

The strongest relationships aren't built on constant excitement or grand displays. They're grounded in simplicity. When two people feel seen, heard, and cared for, their connection naturally deepens. Complications often arise when we add layers of ego, unspoken expectations, or power dynamics. But when we return to the basics—listening with empathy, showing up with kindness, offering consistent care—relationships thrive. We don't need to be in agreement at all times or avoid conflict at all costs. We simply need to hold space for each other with respect and compassion.

At the heart of every meaningful connection is a simple truth: We're here to walk beside one another, to grow, to support, and to share in the beauty and mess of life. True connection like this doesn't have to be complicated. Building relationships that nourish us simply requires our authenticity and care.

Take a moment today to reflect on your most important relationships. Are they nourished by care, understanding, and presence or clouded by complexity and control? Let go of what doesn't serve connection. Return to the basics: Be present, listen deeply, and show care. That's where love and trust will truly begin to grow.

Starting today, how can you simplify and strengthen one relationship in your life?

REVENGE IS EXPENSIVE

Revenge is a debt you don't need to collect. Karma has already sent the invoice and will settle the balance.

Seeking revenge often drains more energy than whatever justice we thought it might restore. While the desire for payback can feel valid in the moment, it rarely delivers the peace we expect. Instead, revenge prolongs pain, keeping us tethered to the very person or situation we want to be free from.

Letting go and releasing your need for some type of justice isn't weakness. It's wisdom. You're making a choice to protect your energy, your joy, and your future. Life has a remarkable way of balancing the scales in due time. And the more you focus on your own healing and growth, the less power the past holds over you.

Choosing peace over retaliation doesn't let others off the hook—it simply takes the hook out of your hand.

The next time you feel the pull toward revenge, pause and ask yourself: *Is pursuing this worth my peace of mind?* Shift your focus inward. Trust that life handles what you don't need to carry. Let peace lead, and watch your freedom expand.

What grudge are you holding that's costing you more than it's giving? Are you ready to let it go?

BREAK FREE FROM COMFORT

Don't let your comfort zone keep you from embracing all life has to offer.

Comfort feels safe—familiar, predictable, easy. But comfort can also keep us small. When we stay in the same routines, avoid the unknown, or stick to what's easy, we may feel secure, yes, but we're also limiting what we can experience.

Growth doesn't come from what you already know but from what you're brave enough to explore. The moment you step outside your comfort zone, you stretch what's possible. You discover new parts of yourself. Your borders expand. You tap into potential you didn't even know was there. Yes, the unfamiliar is uncomfortable, but that discomfort is often the doorway to clarity, confidence, and deeper fulfillment.

Life isn't meant to be survived in safety—it's meant to be fully lived in courage.

Challenge yourself to do one thing today that stretches your margins. Say yes to something that scares you a little. You don't need to leap, but you do need to move. Everything you want to grow into is waiting just beyond where you feel most at ease.

Where in your life have you stayed comfortable for too long? What would happen if you stepped beyond it?

YOU FOR YOU

It's always been you versus you—
or better yet, you for you.

You may have believed at various points that your circumstances, other people's opinions, or even luck held more power over your life than you did, that external forces controlled your destiny. But every meaningful life change begins within—not with others but with *you.*

Change starts with a choice. Even in your lowest moments, you're the one who decides to keep going, to grow, to expand. It's easy to view your struggles as a battle—*you versus you*—but that mind-set will only deepen the divide.

When you stop fighting yourself and start standing *with* yourself—*you for you*—you will notice a shift. You'll stop tearing down and begin rebuilding. You'll realize that you don't need to conquer who you have been but instead support who you're becoming.

That choice? That inner alliance? It's the spark that will start a quiet, powerful revolution from within.

If you've been stuck in self-doubt, comparison, or blame, take a moment to look inward. Your journey doesn't require proving your worth to the world. Your only goal is to prove your love to yourself. Choose to be on your own team.

What would shift in your life if you started working *for* instead of *against* yourself?

MARCH 5

THE POWER OF SERVICE

Purpose and contentment come when we choose to serve humanity.

If you live long enough, one truth will become clear: Fulfillment doesn't come from personal gain alone. We experience true fulfillment through the lives we touch, the encouragement we offer, and the compassion we extend.

Whether you're guiding others, lending a hand, or simply showing kindness in a moment that matters, these acts build a better world—and they build a better you. Serving others brings about a remarkable equation: Every small gesture rooted in service ripples outward . . . and then back inward as well. That energy is amplified and then returned back to you.

Serving others isn't just a noble ideal. It's a guaranteed path to deep purpose, meaningful connection, and lasting impact.

Seek opportunities to serve others with kindness, compassion, and selflessness. Look for ways to positively impact your community, whether through small gestures or grand efforts. Understand that being of service will not only benefit those around you but will also bring a sense of fulfillment and purpose to your life. Do your actions reflect your commitment to lifting others up and contributing to a better world?

What one way can you try to serve someone else today?

HOW TO BE READY

If you rush into something before you're ready, you may stumble over lessons you weren't prepared to learn.

In a world that glorifies speed, it's easy to think we have to act fast or we risk being left behind. But leaping too soon often leads to unnecessary struggle. True growth responds to preparation, not pressure. And readiness is about more than feeling confident. You must actually be in alignment. There's a big difference between waiting aimlessly and preparing intentionally.

Waiting for readiness isn't the same as standing still. It's the quiet, deliberate work of preparing—mentally, emotionally, and spiritually—for the moment you know is coming. You lay the foundation so that when the opportunity appears, you're not scrambling to start. You're already standing, ready to step forward.

Don't confuse urgency with purpose. When you honor the timing of your own unfolding, you step into opportunity with clarity, strength, and grace.

Before rushing into your next pursuit, pause and ask: *Am I stepping forward because of the fear of missing out, or am I stepping forward from a place of true readiness?* Let preparation be your power. Trust that when the time is right, you won't need to force anything. Whatever it is will naturally flow.

What area of your life is calling for preparation rather than speed right now?

WHO OWNS TRUTH?

Facts don't belong to any one of us.
They belong only to the truth.

In an age driven by noise, speed, and constant opinions, it's dangerously easy to confuse conviction with truth. Social media, news cycles, and even daily conversations often become arenas where facts are twisted to fit identity, ideology, or party. But none of us owns truth; it isn't something for us to possess, bend, or weaponize. Real truth demands humility. To honor truth, we must release ego, challenge our assumptions, and stay open to perspectives that stretch our understanding.

Real truth comes into clarity when we stop defending what we think we know and become willing to listen, to question, to learn. Owning the truth is less about claiming authority and more about cultivating clarity, respect, and discernment. It requires patience, emotional maturity, and the courage to listen even when it's uncomfortable.

Truth has no allegiance—it stands alone, waiting for recognition, not validation.

Before rushing to prove your point, pause and ask: *Am I defending my pride, or am I discovering what's real?* Choose curiosity over certainty, and let truth guide your growth.

What truth are you brave enough to seek—even if it unravels what you believed about yourself or the world around you?

THE GIFT OF WISDOM

The greatest gift you can give isn't the answer.
It's the wisdom to find the answer.

Whether you're a parent, mentor, teacher, or friend, your role isn't to fix everything. Your role is to create the space for someone else to think, question, and grow. At first, you might feel the urge to protect, to provide a solution, to shield them from struggle. But real guidance doesn't come from solving. It comes from empowering.

When you help another person learn how to think critically, feel deeply, and navigate uncertainty, you give them a gift far more lasting than any shortcut. You give them the ability to look inward, to seek out wisdom. Wisdom isn't handed down, but you can help others cultivate it through experience, reflection, and the quiet encouragement to find their own way.

Resist the urge to jump in with solutions in the various interactions in your life. Instead, ask questions that inspire curiosity. Offer support that empowers decision-making. Trust that another person's path to wisdom may look different, but it will be theirs. That's the best gift we can give those we love—the confidence and ability to find answers on their own.

What kind of wisdom are you passing on to another individual—and will it guide them when you're not there?

THE STRENGTH IN ASKING

Asking for help isn't weakness. True power lives in vulnerability and community.

You may have picked up the misconception somewhere along the way that silence equals strength—that holding it all together on your own is what makes a person resilient. And you've done it: You've carried heavy burdens alone, stayed silent when you were in pain, isolated when you needed others.

But real strength lives in our willingness to *share* the weight of life with others. Asking for help isn't weakness; it's wisdom. Asking doesn't mean we're giving up. We're letting someone in to help us succeed. Choosing to be vulnerable means you are breaking yourself *open*—to support, to connection, to healing, to growth.

You don't have to carry your burdens alone. The moment you say, "I need help," you open a door—to love, to guidance, and to the strength and wisdom of others who've walked similar roads. You're not meant to do this alone.

Take inventory of what you've been carrying alone. Ask yourself: *What is one place in my life where I can ask for support?* Make the call. Send the message. And then speak your truth.

What part of your life is too heavy to carry alone? Are you brave enough to ask for help today?

ANCHORED IN THE PRESENT

The saying "Be here now" is easier than you may think. There's nowhere else you can truly be.

You may think that presence is something you have to work toward or earn—through meditation, stillness, or the perfect moment. But the truth is, you're already here. Your mind might race ahead to what's next or wander back to what was, but your body never leaves the now. That's your doorway to presence—when you stop running from what already is, right here and right now.

Presence isn't something you achieve—it's something you return to. It's as simple as noticing your breath, the ground beneath your feet, or the sound around you. No need to fix or change anything. Just pause. Feel. Let yourself arrive in the moment. That's presence—accessible anytime, anywhere. Peace will rise. Clarity will return. And suddenly, the moment you tried to catch will catch you instead.

When you feel overwhelmed, close your eyes and place a hand on your heart. Feel your breath. Allow yourself to be here fully and freely in this moment.

What might shift in your life if you allowed the present moment, just as it is, to be enough?

THE POWER OF COMMITMENT

Interest is curious. Commitment is relentless.

There's a subtle but powerful distinction between being interested in something and being committed to it. Interest shows up when it's convenient—when conditions are ideal, when motivation is high. But commitment? Commitment shows up when you continue to do something hard, when it's uncomfortable, when no one is watching.

Commitment doesn't ask for permission or perfect timing. Commitment creates its own momentum. It turns intention into action and dreams into reality. The truth is, you won't always *feel* ready (even when you really are). You won't dive into each new pursuit with total clarity and confidence.

But if you're committed, you'll take that next step. Because commitment isn't passive. It doesn't rely on circumstances; it relies on choice. It isn't a fleeting fancy. Commitment is powerful. It's the bridge between who you are and who you're becoming.

Ask yourself: *Am I interested, or am I committed?* Then take one bold step that proves your answer. Don't wait for the perfect conditions to begin whatever it is you feel called to do. Create them.

Where in your life is interest holding you back, and what would shift if you chose full commitment instead?

THE FREEDOM OF NON-JUDGMENT

When you stop judging others, you free yourself to live your own truth—no comparisons, no shame.

Judgment often acts as a mirror, reflecting the very insecurities, fears, or expectations we haven't addressed within ourselves. Judgment can feel like control, but it quietly cages both the person being judged and the one doing the judging. Real freedom begins when we choose to see others without the need to categorize or critique them. That mindset shift invites deeper understanding, both of ourselves and those around us. When we replace judgment with awareness, we release the pressure to conform, impress, or defend. We stop measuring our worth against others and begin living from a place of truth.

Non-judgment doesn't mean indiscriminate agreement with others or their actions. It means you're choosing presence instead—meeting each moment, each person, and each version of yourself with openness rather than resistance. That spirit of non-judgment will bring peace. And that peace will make room for real growth.

As you move through your day, notice when judgment arises inside you. Don't criticize yourself. Get curious instead. Replace the urge to label with a commitment to learning. Let understanding guide your interactions, and watch as your inner world softens in return.

What part of your life would feel lighter if you released judgment and replaced it with acceptance?

THE VALUE OF TRUE FRIENDSHIP

A person doesn't need many friends.
One true friend is all it takes.

Friendship isn't about how many people are in your life—it's about the depth of connection you share. One friend who truly sees you, supports you, and stands beside you in both joy and struggle is worth more than a hundred acquaintances.

Real friendship isn't loud or flashy. It's steady. Quiet. Honest. It's the person who shows up—not just when it's easy or fun but also when it's hard, when you're hurting, and when words fall short. You don't need a crowd to feel loved. One person who knows your heart and holds it with care, one genuine bond that offers peace, trust, and strength, is more fulfilling than a roomful of surface-level relationships.

Sometimes, just one other soul in sync with yours is all it takes to remind you that you're not alone.

Who in your life has shown up with real loyalty and care, particularly when you were down? Don't chase more relationships. Deepen what already brings connection. Nurture the friendships that truly feed your soul.

**Name the one person you can always count on.
How will you honor that friendship today?**

EMPOWERING INDEPENDENCE

Real transformation and growth come when we let go and trust our loved ones to make their own choices.

One of the hardest lessons in life is letting go. This is especially true in the parent-child dynamic. Our instinct from the time of our child's birth is to protect, guide, and hold on tightly. But real love includes trust—and that trust empowers children to grow into their strength, values, and purpose.

The same holds true for any relationship in which we serve as a guiding force. When we let go, we step back just enough to allow our loved ones to *step forward*. We allow space in that person's journey for them to take their own steps.

Growth often happens not in our grip but in our grace. And when we trust those we've helped nurture to find their own way, we will witness something beautiful.

Reflect on your role as a parent or mentor. Are you trying to control the outcome, or are you creating space for learning, failure, and growth? Show those you are guiding that you trust them—through your words, actions, and even silence. Support their steps without steering every movement. Let your love be the foundation, not a fence.

Where in your guidance can you loosen your grip and rely on the foundation you've helped build?

THE WEIGHT OF UNCHECKED ANGER

Left unchecked, anger can turn a brief moment into a lasting regret.

Anger often arrives quickly—loud, hot, hurried—but its consequences can linger far longer than the moment itself. Many of us have let frustration speak for us, only to be left with regret and fractured trust that takes a great deal of time to earn back. Once angry words are spoken or swift actions are taken, they can't be undone.

Don't underestimate the power in the pause. Between the swell of anger and how we act on it lies a small but sacred space. In that space, we have a choice. A single breath can shift everything. When we learn to pause, we protect not only our relationships but also our peace and integrity.

Anger itself isn't wrong. To feel anger is to be human. But without a mindful response, anger can be destructive. When we meet anger with awareness, we allow anger to become a teacher instead of a weapon.

The next time anger rises up inside you, pause. Take a few breaths. Ask yourself: *Is this response aligned with who I truly want to be?* Then choose calm. That single moment of reflection can prevent a lifetime of regret.

What might change in your relationships if you paused long enough to let peace speak before anger could?

THE TRUE COST OF MENTAL OVERLOAD

If you're constantly thinking or dreaming about work, you're still working, just without the paycheck.

You may close your laptop, walk away from your desk, and silence the notifications, but if your thoughts are still looping around deadlines, decisions, or what's next, you haven't really stopped working. Mental overload is silent, sneaky, and suffocating. It wears the mask of commitment but ends up draining your creativity, your presence, and your peace.

Being ambitious isn't the same as being consumed. True high performance requires recovery. Just like a muscle grows in rest, your clarity and energy rebuild in the pause. When you reclaim your mind, you not only feel better; you also think better, lead better, and live better.

Start honoring your off switch. Create a clear boundary between work and well-being. Set rituals that remind your nervous system it's safe to relax—whether it's a walk, gentle stretching, music, or silence. You're not slacking when you unplug. You're sustaining your power.

As you get ready for bed tonight, ask yourself: *Have I given my mind permission to rest?* If not, release the mental weights. You deserve peace in the present—not just when the job is done. Because your well-being is worth protecting every day.

How much energy are you sacrificing without you even realizing it?

THE LIGHT KNOWS THE WAY

Part of you fears the dark, and another part of you holds the light. Let the light lead.

We all go through moments—mentally, emotionally, spiritually—when fear, doubt, and pain try to convince us that we're lost. That we'll never figure out what comes next. That we'll always struggle. That peace just isn't meant for us.

In those moments, it's easy to forget that part of us remains untouched by the noise and the negativity. Quiet but steady, this small inner flame never goes out. It is the light of our truth. Our inner clarity. Our compass. It doesn't shout at us, demanding attention. It gently calls us back to center. And every time we choose to follow it, even amid uncertainty, we uncover a strength we didn't know we had.

Fear might be loud, but the quiet light within always knows the way forward. Trust your inner light. Even when the path ahead is dim, it is there, guiding you home.

When you find yourself in emotional darkness or uncertainty, pause and turn inward. Take a deep breath and ask: *What does the calm, wise, steady part of me know?* Whether it's nudging you to rest, speak up, change your environment, or keep going, let it lead you forward.

When fear clouds your vision, how can you choose to follow the light within?

YOU DETERMINE YOUR IDENTITY

Your identity isn't shaped by your experiences but by the person you've become because of them.

Life will challenge you, stretch you, even break you open. But that pain doesn't define you. You aren't the difficult childhood, the financial mistakes, the failed relationships. You are what you choose to do with those experiences. Every hardship carries a lesson. Every win brings with it responsibility. Every season offers you a chance not only to survive but to *transform*. You are not the difficult events you've been through. You are the strength you've found inside them.

What makes you *you*? You're made up of your experiences. You are the choices you made when things got tough. You are the compassion you learned after being hurt. You are the resilience you built when life didn't go your way. You are the humility you embraced after failure.

You are not your wounds—you are your healing. You aren't your failures—you are how you overcome. You aren't your history—you are the author of what comes next.

Don't let your past confine or define you. Instead of asking, *What did I go through?* ask, *Who did I become?* That answer will reveal your truth.

Think about a time that challenged your identity. How did you rise up in that moment to become more of who you truly are?

OWNING YOUR CHOICES

The only way to move on from your mistakes is to own your choices and grow from what you've learned.

It's easy to convince ourselves that avoiding responsibility for our actions might ease the sting of past mistakes. But real growth begins with ownership, not avoidance or guilt. When we take responsibility without shame, we stop being victims of our past and become students of it. Mistakes turn into lessons. Regret becomes insight. Owning our choices doesn't mean excusing them—it means taking accountability, learning from them, and then doing better the next time.

Reliving the past will never bring healing. We truly heal when we grow beyond the past. When we face our truth with courage, we reclaim our power. Responsibility becomes a tool for transformation rather than an instrument of punishment. And we can begin to move forward—this time wiser, stronger, and more grounded in who we are becoming.

Think of a mistake that still lingers in your heart. Instead of avoiding it, be present in this moment and own it. Ask yourself: *What truth do I need to accept? Where might I need to forgive myself or apologize to someone else? What lesson can I carry forward?* Let this reflection mark the beginning of your next chapter.

What one truth are you ready to own today so you can reclaim your power?

STICK TO THE PLAN

When the pain of unhealthy habits finally outweighs the effort to change, sticking to the plan becomes easier.

For many of us, there comes a time when the weight of unhealthy habits becomes too much to carry. At first, those habits might feel like relief—something to lean on in stressful times: one too many trips through the drive-thru, night after night of staying up late watching TV, general habits of carelessness with your health. But eventually, these things cost more than they give. They rob your energy, confidence, and clarity—begging the question: *Is this activity worth how it makes me feel?*

When the discomfort of staying in your habits outweighs the pain of growing beyond them, commitment to change becomes easier. The plan toward a better you stops feeling like a chore and starts feeling like freedom. Sticking to a healthy lifestyle isn't about perfection—it's about remembering what you've already outgrown. And choosing, every day, not to return to what once held you back.

Take a moment to reflect: *What habit is quietly stealing my energy or peace? What truth am I finally ready to face?* Use that awareness as fuel. Choose the plan instead of the pain. Let your discomfort become the push that moves you forward.

What one step can you take today to honor the life you're ready to live?

LEAVE ONE WINDOW OPEN

Sometimes one open window is enough to let the light find you while you heal.

Healing doesn't always arrive with clarity or certainty. More often, healing begins with a quiet choice—to keep your heart open, just a little.

When life feels overwhelming, your instinct might be to shut everything out. To protect, to retreat, to close every door so you can stay safe and survive. Even in those moments, try to leave one window open—a single space where light can reach you, a crack in the armor, a whisper to the world that you're still here, still willing, still becoming. That open window doesn't need to fix everything. It is simply a reminder that something good still exists—that warmth, connection, and peace are still possible.

That window is your quiet *yes* to life. Your permission to hope. And your proof that healing doesn't have to be loud.

> You don't have to choose between being completely open and closing yourself off. You can protect your peace and still stay open . . . even if only a little. Leave space for the light to find you, however small, however uncertain. Sometimes just one window can brighten the whole room.

Where in your life can you soften just enough to let something good back in?

YOU HOLD THE KEY TO YOUR HEALTH

You hold the key to your health and well-being. No one else can turn it for you.

It's easy to wait it out when it comes to our wellness. To hope that someone else will have the answers. That we'll come up with a new plan. That we'll find the perfect coach, partner, or motivation. But here's the truth: The key to your health is already in your hands.

Your health—physical, emotional, mental, and spiritual—is *your* responsibility. No one else can unlock the door for you. Others can guide you, inspire you, and support you, but only you can make the move. Only you can turn the key. That doesn't mean you're on this journey alone. But you do have to approach choices with intention—what you consume, how you move, how you rest, and how you speak to yourself.

Every choice you make is a turn of the key. Every moment you decide to show up for yourself, no matter how big or small, will bring you closer to unlocking a life of strength, clarity, and peace.

Take one bold step today that says: *I choose my well-being*. Stop waiting for permission—this is your life, your body, your power.

What part of your well-being have you been handing over to someone else? How can you take it back today?

THE QUIET TEST OF INTEGRITY

Would you choose the same path if no one were watching? The quiet test of integrity reveals the real you.

Your integrity isn't defined by how others see you. True integrity is revealed by what you choose when no one else is looking. The real test doesn't happen under a spotlight—it happens in silence. Your core values speak loudest in those private moments when a shortcut seems easier, when a small lie might smooth things over, when no praise is on the line. True integrity isn't about performance or perfection. It's personal and deeply rooted in your core values.

When lies go unchecked, do you still choose honesty?

Do you do what's right, even when wrong is rewarded?

Do you hold firm to your convictions when there's nothing to gain but self-respect?

These quiet, seemingly small decisions become the bedrock of your character. They shape how you show up for yourself and for others. And in the long run, these consistent, often unnoticed actions will embody your strength and authenticity.

The next time you need to make a decision, ask yourself: *Would I make this choice if I knew no one would ever find out?* Let that answer guide your steps. Integrity isn't measured by recognition or validation but by truth and self-awareness.

What silent decision will you make today to strengthen the foundation of who you truly are?

INFINITE LOVE

There's more than enough love to cover the entire world and reach beyond the stars.

Love isn't finite. It's not something we can run out of. Even more, it's something we rise *into*. Love isn't stored in limited supply or measured by its scarcity. The more we give love, the more it grows. Yet so often, we withhold love. We are guarded, cautious, waiting for the "right" time or fearing it won't be reciprocated. But love was never meant to be earned. It was meant to be *given*.

Real love—pure, unconditional love—doesn't shrink when challenged. It doesn't falter when unreturned. It keeps going. It transcends ego, fear, and pain. It reaches across divides and softens what hurt has hardened. Love is the quiet strength behind forgiveness, the force that fuels compassion, and the bridge to connection. It lives within all of us, waiting to be chosen and shared.

The world doesn't need more perfection. It needs more love—and more people willing to love even when it's hard, even when it's vulnerable, even when it's not convenient.

Don't wait for the right conditions to express love. Give it freely today. Speak it, show it, embody it. One act of love can change a moment. Many acts of love can change the world.

Where is your love waiting to be unleashed?

VULNERABILITY IS THE GATEWAY

Love heals all—except the wounds
we refuse to reveal.

At one point or another, many of us have believed that love alone could mend a situation. But over time, a deeper truth comes to light—love can only heal what it's allowed to touch. We often hide our wounds behind resilience, silence, or a smile, hoping that love will somehow reach what we've buried, what we're too fearful to allow another to witness. But love can't heal what it's not invited to see.

Whether it's in a romantic relationship, a friendship, a situation with a family member, or the love we offer ourselves, healing begins with honesty. The moment we say, "This hurt me," we create space, not for love to fix or erase an issue but to bear witness to, soothe, and slowly heal and transform.

Vulnerability isn't weakness—it's the gateway. And when we open up, love not only shows up; it moves in and takes up residence.

What pain have you been hiding from those who love you most? Take one step toward vulnerability—share a truth, ask for support, or write down how you're feeling, just for yourself. Love is ready to meet you if you're willing to open the door.

What healing might begin if you stopped hiding your pain?

BUILT, NOT BORN

Greatness isn't born from ease—it's built by those who turn what they have into what they need.

You don't need perfect conditions to create something extraordinary. You need hunger. You need heart. You need the willingness to work with what's in front of you—and the vision to see beyond it.

Greatness doesn't come gift-wrapped. It's carved from discomfort, from trying when quitting would be easier, from refusing to let lack define your potential. Those who rise aren't the ones who start with everything. They're the ones who *use* everything. They turn every setback, every flaw, every ounce of pain into fuel.

You can't wait for the stars to align. You must recognize the imperfection around you and still choose to build anyway—with steady hands, clarity, and the kind of quiet determination that keeps showing up long before anyone takes notice and well after the crowd has stopped watching.

Look at what's in your hands—not at what's missing, but at what's *possible*. Let your grit do the heavy lifting. Let your vision light the way. You have enough to begin.

What part of your life are you ready to stop waiting on and start building from today?

BREAKING SELF-IMPOSED LIMITS

Saying "I can't" reveals the limits you've set for yourself rather than your true abilities.

Most of the time, when we say "I can't," what we're actually saying is "I won't." We aren't confronting a lack of ability. We're facing a self-built barrier made of fear, doubt, or past conditioning. We label something impossible rather than risk failure.

But the truth? Many of these so-called limits aren't real. They're self-imposed. You were never meant to live inside a box of your own making. You were meant to stretch, to rise, to evolve. Growth doesn't come from playing it safe—it comes when you step beyond the edge of what you *think* you can do and break through those self-imposed limits.

The moment you replace "I can't" with "I will," you reclaim your power. You shift from limitation to liberation, and you stop shrinking and start becoming.

Start paying attention to the language you use with yourself. The next time you hear yourself say or think "I can't," pause and ask: *Is it actually true that I can't, or is that phrase just familiar?* Then take one bold step beyond the familiar.

What might open up if you tried doing what you've been telling yourself you can't do?

THE POWER OF THE PRESENT

A better tomorrow is forged today. Fixate on the future, and you lose both.

Dreaming big fuels our ambition. Those dreams inspire, motivate, and propel us to chase after what matters to us. But becoming obsessed with what's next often disconnects us from what matters most—*this* moment.

There's nothing wrong with chasing milestones, but believing that fulfillment lives just beyond the next achievement can become an obsession. Instead, each time you pause, breathe, and engage with the present, you can discover the clarity, peace, and purpose already within reach. The present isn't just preparation for the future—it's the foundation. It's where our intentions turn into action and transformation takes root.

When you're grounded in today, fully present and engaged, tomorrow becomes a natural extension of your growth, not a destination to chase. Live here. Act now. That's how you shape what comes next.

Bring your attention back to the present. What one small, intentional step can you take today to strengthen your foundation? Whether it's a mindful breath, a conversation, or a bold decision, don't trade today for a tomorrow that hasn't arrived. Presence is your greatest tool for building a life of meaning, balance, and direction.

Your future is shaped in this very moment. How will you choose to live it?

CORE DESIRE

A true core desire isn't found outside yourself. It already exists within you, waiting to be realized.

You don't have to search the world to discover what truly moves you. Your deepest desires already live within you. But it takes stillness and courage to uncover them.

When your energy is spent chasing approval, status, or someone else's version of success, you'll always feel a step behind. That's because external goals, while shiny, rarely satisfy the soul. True fulfillment comes from tuning in instead of looking out. True fulfillment is found when you listen to the quiet voice that speaks up only when you stop performing, stop comparing, and start trusting yourself.

When you honor your core desires—the ones born of authenticity, not expectation—everything changes. Your motivation becomes sustainable. Your direction becomes clear. And your actions carry more meaning because they're fueled by who you are, not who you think you need to be.

Pause and ask: *What do I truly want—not what others expect or what looks impressive, but what feels true to me?* Let that desire guide your next move.

What longing has been quietly waiting inside you?
What would happen if you let it speak?

THE SIGN OF A CALLING

If you would do a task without pay and feel fulfilled, chances are it's your calling, not just a job.

A unique clarity comes when we realize we're doing something not for prestige, pay, or pats on the back but because it lights something inside us. We've all experienced that feeling of being fully present and energized by an activity for no reason other than it being in total alignment with our true self. It's a feeling that can't be manufactured or mistaken.

Jobs may pay the bills, but callings feed the soul. They leave you feeling whole rather than hollow. And although we might not always get paid for our calling (at least not right away), the fulfillment of embracing it is worth more than any paycheck.

That quiet pull, that spark of passion? That's your soul speaking, reminding you of who you are and why you're here. Follow it. That's where you'll find meaning and purpose.

Ask yourself honestly: *What would I continue to do even if no one paid me to do it or noticed?* That answer is a signpost pointing to your calling. Don't ignore it. Instead, nurture it. Create space for it to bloom. Even small steps toward your purpose can lead to a more meaningful, joyful existence.

What calling is quietly asking for your attention? Are you ready to answer it?

SHOW UP FOR YOURSELF

Show up for yourself—and let your
life be the proof that you did.

How you show up each day is a direct reflection of what you believe—about your worth, your strength, and your future. Empowering beliefs lead to intentional action. They help you make choices with clarity, set meaningful boundaries, and take steps that are aligned with who you're becoming.

But when limiting beliefs sneak in—those beliefs rooted in fear, doubt, or past wounds—your actions tend to shrink. You delay. You overthink. You settle. True transformation begins not in massive shifts but in subtle awareness—noticing the story, questioning its truth, and then choosing to write a new one.

When you consistently show up for yourself—through discipline, care, and alignment—life will meet you there. The results may not be instant, but they will come, quietly validating every step you dare to take.

Ask yourself today: *What belief is leading me?* Then act in a way that honors the person you're becoming, not the version you've outgrown. Whether it's a boundary, a breath, or a bold move, do it with intention. You're not just living—you're becoming.

What will your actions today say about what you truly believe you deserve?

APRIL

APRIL 1

THE RESPONSIBILITY OF WISDOM

True wisdom is living as if someone else's tomorrow depends on your life today.

Wisdom isn't measured by what you know—your knowledge, your intellect. Wisdom is revealed in *how you live*. Every action, every word, every quiet decision leaves a mark, not just on your path but on the paths of those walking beside and behind you.

Whether you realize it or not, someone is watching. Someone is listening. Someone is learning how to move forward by witnessing your life. Living with wisdom means living with awareness. It means recognizing that your influence reaches further than your own life. This doesn't mean you're expected to be perfect. Wisdom asks only that you be present. Be intentional. Choose the path of integrity, not just for your benefit but because of the light it will shine into others' storms.

This is the responsibility that comes with wisdom: to know that your strength could be someone else's shelter, that your resilience might inspire another to rise. At every step of your journey, wisdom asks, "Who might this help?"

Pause and take a breath. Ask yourself: *What message is my life sending today?* Let your example become a source of encouragement, not just for yourself but for someone else who might need it.

Who might be waiting for your example so they can take their next step?

LET YOUR LIGHT SHINE

Get out of your own way. Your light can only shine when you stop standing in its path.

Sometimes your biggest obstacle isn't the world—it's you. The doubts you feed and the stories you replay stand in your way. The hesitation keeps you stuck. You weren't born to be diluted, dimmed, or shut off. But somewhere along the way, you started believing the fears more than the blaze inside you.

Like clouds covering the sun, those thoughts don't erase your light—they only block it. The good news? You can move them. You can shift the pattern, question the belief, and make space for brilliance to come through.

Your light doesn't need fixing—it needs freedom, a clear path to shine through. And that begins the moment you decide to stop standing in your own way.

Notice what thoughts, habits, or fears are clouding your shine. Then take one step—small but clear—to move them aside. You were never meant to live in shadow. You were meant to shine brightly.

What's one way you've been standing in the way of your own light—and what will you do today to let that light through?

THE PARADOX OF TIME

Days can feel endless, yet the years pass in a flash.

Time plays tricks on us. Some days feel impossibly long—packed with stress, repetition, waiting. Yet somehow, the months vanish. The years slip by. One moment you're navigating today's grind, and the next you're wondering where the last decade went.

That's the paradox of time. It moves slow in the moment and impossibly fast in memory. And in that contrast is a truth we often overlook: Each seemingly ordinary day matters more than we realize. Every routine, every conversation, every pause—they all stack up to build a life. If we sleepwalk through the moments, we miss the meaning. But when we live with presence, even the longest days begin to glow with significance.

Life isn't measured only by milestones. It's written in the ordinary moments we choose to fully inhabit.

Don't wait for special occasions to be truly awake. This day—the one you're living right now—is part of your legacy. Slow down. Savor the seconds. Let presence be your gift to time. Because the way you live your moments is the way you shape your years.

What would change if you treated today not as something to "get through" but as a moment you'll one day wish you could revisit?

THE ILLUSION OF LIMITS

The only obstacles standing between you and success are the excuses you choose to believe.

Most of the limits you face aren't external. They're limits you've accepted without questioning where they came from: "I'm not ready." "I don't have what it takes." "Now's not the time." These thoughts feel real, but they're often fear in disguise. When you peel back the layers, you discover this truth: Your ability isn't holding you back; the story you've been telling yourself about your ability is.

Every excuse is a wall, but every action is a sledgehammer. The moment you stop waiting for permission or perfection and start moving forward—however imperfectly—those walls will begin to crumble. Your potential isn't waiting to be found. It's waiting for you to claim it. What you believe about yourself will either limit you or lead you.

Choose to believe in your ability to rise, even when the evidence hasn't fully caught up yet.

Choose one excuse you've outgrown. Question it. Replace it with one small, bold step in the direction of your vision. You don't need to have it all figured out. You just need to begin.

What excuse have you been believing—and what truth will you replace it with today?

SANCTUARY OF STRENGTH

The gym is more than a place to work out—it's a sanctuary for growth.

The gym is more than four walls filled with weights and mirrors—it's a sacred space of transformation. It's where distractions fade and the present moment sharpens. Where each lift, stretch, or stride isn't just physical—it's symbolic.

A rep against doubt.

A step toward discipline.

A breath into resilience.

But the space becomes sacred only when we treat it with intention. When we respect the energy we bring, the effort others give, and the body we're entrusted to strengthen, the gym becomes a place of evolution instead of ego.

Whether you're chasing strength, peace, or purpose, the gym is a sanctuary when you show up with presence. And in that presence, you don't just build muscle—you build mind-set.

The next time you enter the gym, leave comparison at the door. Train not only for the purpose of looking strong, but *being* strong—in spirit, in focus, in integrity. Every drop of sweat is a choice to rise.

How will you transform your workout into a ritual that strengthens not just your body but also your being?

THE QUIET HEART OF ABUNDANCE

True abundance reveals itself not in what we possess, but in the quiet whisper of peace.

You've been taught that abundance is a finish line—something to earn, gather, or prove. This lie tells you that you'll finally be satisfied when you buy a bigger house, upgrade your social circle, or achieve the world's next great physical feat. But real abundance doesn't shout with numbers or flash with things. It whispers through peace. You find abundance in your heart when you no longer panic over what's missing or compare yourself to someone else's measure of success.

Abundance shows up in the stillness and carries you forward. You realize you already have enough to breathe, to love, to rise. Realizing you have enough is not settling. It's seeing and acknowledging the quiet wealth that lives in your breath, your relationships, your commitment to growth, and your ability to begin again.

You can chase more and still feel empty. Or you can stand still, feel what's already here, and be filled.

Shift your focus from lack to presence. List what you once longed for that's now part of your life. Let that recognition fill you with peace and gratitude.

How would your life change if you believed that true wealth isn't found in your hands, but in your heart?

THE FLOW OF KINDNESS

Kindness flows naturally when
you rise above your ego.

Kindness isn't weakness. Kindness is wisdom in motion. Yet often our ego gets in the way, whispering, "They don't deserve it," or "You'll look weak," or "What's in it for you?"

While ego thrives on separation, kindness thrives on connection. When we rise above the need to win, to impress, to control, we tap into something much deeper—our shared humanity. Kindness, then, isn't a performance. It's not a transaction. And it certainly isn't weak. Kindness is a choice made out of presence, humility, and courage. It's a quiet offering of warmth in a world that often feels cold.

And the beauty of choosing kindness? Kindness has a ripple effect. One small act can shift the energy in a room, soften someone's defenses, or even inspire change where nothing else could.

Pay attention to the moments today when your ego wants to lead. Instead of asserting, choose understanding. Instead of judging, choose compassion. Let kindness flow, not as an effort, but as a return to who you really are. Because when ego steps aside, love—and change—step in.

What would happen if kindness became your default response?

EMPOWER, DON'T ENABLE

Empower others rather than enabling them.

Support doesn't mean doing everything for someone—stepping in, fixing, providing. Support means believing in the other person's ability to grow. Yet in our desire to help, we often rob others of the very process that will build their strength.

True empowerment is teaching, not rescuing. It's saying, "I believe you can do this," and then giving the person tools instead of a shortcut. Solving a problem for someone may bring temporary relief, but lasting transformation comes when you empower and equip them. Empowerment helps others discover their own resourcefulness, make wise choices, and build resilience. The goal isn't dependence. The goal is self-leadership.

When you guide instead of carrying, when you're a catalyst rather than a crutch, you show someone they're capable. You build not just results—but also confidence, courage, and the kind of self-trust that lasts far beyond a single moment of help.

Shift your support from providing solutions to offering strength. Share your insights, your guidance, your faith in the other person's potential. True leadership isn't about being the hero; it's about helping others become their own hero.

Where in your life can you step back to empower someone to rise on their own?

THE GIFT OF SENSITIVITY

Creative minds feel deeply. When honored, that sensitivity becomes a powerful source of vision.

Sensitivity often manifests itself in creativity. And this creativity isn't born from numbness. It's born from a depth of emotion. From the courage to feel it all—the awe, the wonder, the ache, the uncertainty. A creative mind doesn't just skim the surface; it dives deep, exploring both light and shadow in our world.

Sensitivity can feel like a burden at times, leaving you vulnerable to doubt and fear. But when you honor it instead of resisting it, it becomes your greatest source of vision. It's the lens that lets you see what others overlook. It's the heartbeat behind every idea, every breakthrough, every act of creation.

Feeling deeply isn't weakness. It's a sacred strength. It's how beauty is born. It's how truth finds its voice. It's how art, innovation, and real connection come alive.

Instead of shielding yourself from your sensitivity, lean into it. Let it sharpen your vision, fuel your creativity, and deepen your connection to the world around you.

How can you honor your sensitivity today and recognize it as the powerful gift it truly is?

THE WISDOM OF ANXIETY

Anxiety is often a sign of misalignment—a gentle nudge to return to the present and find understanding.

Anxiety is often misunderstood. While it can feel overwhelming in the moment—a sense of panic, a lack of control, crippling fear—anxiety isn't always a sign that something is wrong. It may be a signal that something within us is asking for attention.

Many people experience anxiety when they feel out of sync with their values, disconnected from the present, or consumed by a desire to control the uncontrollable. And the more we resist it, the more power anxiety seems to have.

But when we shift from resistance to awareness, something changes. We begin to see anxiety not as the enemy but as a messenger who can guide us to pause, reflect, and realign with what truly matters. You will find clarity and freedom when you stop avoiding anxious feelings and seek understanding of what they're pointing to.

When you feel anxious, don't push the feeling away. Instead, get curious: *What part of me needs attention? Where might I be out of alignment?* Use your breath to ground yourself and gently return to the present. You'll often find clarity hiding beneath the surface.

What might anxiety be trying to tell you? What would it look like to listen to your anxiety instead of fighting it?

APRIL 11

KEEPING PROMISES TO YOURSELF

Discipline is more than a routine. Discipline is your declaration of your self-worth.

Discipline is often seen as rigid or joyless—as if it's just about willpower or forcing yourself to do things you might not want to do. But real discipline is something deeper. It's an act of self-devotion.

Every time you choose to follow through—whether it's waking up early, moving your body, nourishing yourself, or saying no to what no longer serves you—you're affirming something powerful: *I matter. My growth matters. My future is worth the effort.* Discipline isn't about being perfect. It's about *being present*—in your choices, in your commitments, in your journey. It's about showing up when it's not easy. It's about keeping your promises to yourself, not because others are watching but because *you* are watching.

When you keep showing up for yourself, your self-trust builds. Your confidence grows. Your self-respect deepens. That's the true reward.

Look at your daily habits through a new lens: *What part of me am I honoring when I commit to this action?* Let every step you take be a quiet, steady reminder that you are worth the effort.

What's one habit you can reclaim today as a declaration of your worth?

THE STRENGTH OF YOUR EMOTIONS

Staying strong doesn't mean repressing your feelings—it means facing them.

You may have been taught that strength looks like silence, that holding it all together without cracking is what makes you resilient. But real strength has nothing to do with pretending everything's fine or keeping up appearances.

Strength isn't about bottling up pain, denying fear, or hiding behind a mask of composure. True strength shows up when you allow yourself to feel—fully, honestly, without apology. Strength reveals itself when you sit with your sadness instead of running from it, when you admit you're hurting and still choose to move forward. You don't gain power by pushing emotions down but by experiencing them, expressing them, and letting them teach you, guide you, and heal you.

Vulnerability doesn't make you weak. In fact, it's your greatest strength. The most grounded people you'll ever meet are the ones who've allowed themselves to break open and then build back with wisdom instead of walls.

The next time a difficult emotion rises, don't shut it down. Acknowledge it. Name it. Feel it. Then ask what that emotion is trying to show you. Every feeling you face becomes reclaimed strength.

What emotions are you avoiding? What would it take to meet them with honesty instead of resistance?

APRIL 13

BORN TO BRAVE THE SEA

A ship may be safe in harbor, but it was built to brave the open sea.

We often stay where it feels safe—not because we lack courage but because we forget what we're made for. Routines, comfort zones, and predictable paths may bring a sense of control, but they can also become silent prisons. Maybe it's staying in a job that no longer lights you up. Or saying yes to everyone else's needs while ignoring your own. Safety can seduce you into complacency, but purpose calls you forward.

Just like a ship isn't meant to stay docked, we aren't here merely to exist. We're meant to venture, to risk, to grow. The open sea, with all its uncertainty, is where discovery lives. Every wave we face will shape us, strengthen us, and reveal the depth of our resilience.

Staying in the harbor may feel safe, but the real danger lies in never setting sail—never discovering the horizons meant for you. Safety protects in the short term but robs us long term.

If fear or uncertainty has kept you anchored, breathe and push off from the dock. The seas may be unpredictable, but they hold your growth, your purpose, your becoming. You were born to move forward, even when storms come.

What part of your life is ready to leave harbor and sail into possibility?

THE QUIET POWER OF LISTENING

You don't need to speak over others to be heard. Presence, patience, and clarity will amplify your voice better.

You might have convinced yourself that in order to be heard, you must be the loudest voice in the room—that speaking quickly, firmly, or forcefully proves your worth. But what if your real influence lies in your ability to listen? There's a quiet power in the act of listening. That's because listening isn't weak; it's empowering.

Choosing to listen means you want to absorb rather than react, to hold space rather than rush to fill it. Resisting the impulse to interrupt requires emotional maturity. Through inner clarity, you recognize that not everything needs your *opinion*—but everything deserves your *attention*.

When you listen with intention, you create a space for trust, understanding, and connection. You notice what's beneath the words—emotion, meaning, nuance. Real communication happens when you quietly listen and prioritize presence over performance.

In your next conversation, try something radical: Listen without planning your reply. Pause before responding. Let stillness lead. You might be surprised how much more you understand—about others and about yourself.

What might change in your relationships if you listened, not so you could reply, but so you could truly connect?

APRIL 15

THE SHAPE OF LIGHT

The shadow, not the absence of light, gives definition to our brightest moments.

We often try to chase away the darkness—as if the goal is to live only in the light. But the truth is, light means nothing without shadow. Contrast brings clarity. The struggle gives triumph its meaning. The most radiant parts of your life are defined not by perfection but by what you've endured to reach them.

The shadow isn't your enemy. It's your sculptor. It shapes your perspective, sharpens your values, and deepens your appreciation for what you now hold. You see beauty more clearly because you've known the blur of pain. You recognize peace because you've walked through chaos. And it's often in the shadow where your truest strengths are revealed—quiet, steady, and hard-earned.

Without darkness, light has no edge. No definition. No weight. It's the tension between both that makes your story unforgettable.

Don't fear the shadow. Let it reveal the brilliance already within you. Because sometimes your darkest moments give birth to your brightest light.

What moment of light in your life has been shaped by thc shadow that came before it?

RISE WITH INTENTION

Getting out of bed isn't the same as being awake in body and mind—alert, engaged, and truly living.

There are three kinds of people: those who rise and embrace the day, those who stay in bed, and those who go through the motions as if in a trance. You can be out of bed, dressed, and busy and still feel miles from living a life of meaning. It's easy to slip into autopilot, checking boxes without connecting, going through the motions without feeling the joy.

But there's a different way. The shift happens when you choose to rise with intention. When you greet the day not just by waking your body but also by engaging your heart and mind. Life feels alive when we are fully awake in all facets, tuned in, each moment becoming a chance to grow, contribute, and connect.

You weren't made only to exist. You were made to live fully.

Which of the three types of people are you today? Which will you be tomorrow? Choose to rise with purpose. Start each morning by setting one meaningful intention—gratitude, presence, courage—and act on it. Show up for your life.

What intention will help you move from motion to meaning, and how will you live it today?

APRIL 17

MEET YOURSELF HERE

Be yourself—even if you're still learning to love who you see.

The path to self-growth doesn't begin with fixing everything we dislike about ourselves. We take the first step when we accept who we are *right now*. So many of us have stood in front of the mirror, questioning not just our appearance but also our worth—emotionally, mentally, even spiritually. It's easy to believe we have to change before we can love ourselves.

But real transformation doesn't begin with judgment. It begins with grace. The more we accept who we are in this moment, the easier it will be to grow into who we're meant to be. Growth rooted in self-compassion is not only kinder; it's also stronger, deeper, and more lasting than any change fueled by self-criticism.

You don't have to be perfect to be loved and to reach for growth. Meet yourself where you are, and be gentle with yourself as you go.

Pause today and meet yourself exactly where you are. Offer grace instead of judgment. You don't have to have everything figured out to be worthy of love. Accept yourself as you are, and trust that real transformation is just beginning.

What might happen if you stopped striving for perfection and started growing from a place of acceptance instead?

LASTING TRANSFORMATION BEGINS IN THE MIND

Master your mind, and your body will follow.

Although diet culture, "fitfluencers," and the latest nutrition trend may try to convince us otherwise, lasting physical transformation doesn't start with what we eat or how often we exercise. Weight loss is 60 percent mind-set, 30 percent nutrition, and only 10 percent exercise. Lasting health and wellness starts with how we *think*.

You can follow the best, most "proven" nutrition or fitness plan in the world, but if your mind-set is filled with doubt, guilt, quick-fix thinking, or defeatism, progress will stall. Or you may hit a goal—only to gain the weight back and abandon your rigid fitness schedule soon after.

True change begins when you believe you're worthy of feeling good. When your thoughts align with your goals, everything becomes more intentional—your choices, your habits, your self-talk. When your mind leads with clarity and conviction, the body will respond.

Before you change your eating habits or your workouts, ask yourself: *Are my thoughts building the life I want, or are they holding me back? How do I need to shift my mind-set?* Align your inner world, and the outer will follow.

What would happen if you started your health journey with belief in yourself and your worth instead of pressure?

APRIL 19

THE LANGUAGE OF LOVE AND LAUGHTER

When love and humor meet, they create a sacred bond of healing and deepened connection.

Laughter rooted in love can act as a powerful bridge between souls. Shared laughter is a form of recognition. It's a way of communicating, "I feel safe with you, and I can be myself. I see you, and you see me." Love wrapped in humor lightens the burdens of life in this world. It allows us to meet one another in the middle of struggles with a smile, turn tension into tenderness, and remember joy even in difficulty.

Some of the most profound moments of intimacy are born not from deep conversations but from shared laughter—those unfiltered moments when two people forget the world and simply exist and experience life together. It's a dance of joy, a rhythm of knowing, a quiet reminder that even through the storms, lightness can live between two hearts.

Don't underestimate the healing power of humor in your closest relationships. Lean into joy. Embrace those moments that make you both laugh out loud. Beyond the life-giving humor of the moment, you experience the gift of being real, being present, and being connected.

Where in your relationships can more laughter create deeper love, and how can you invite in that joy today?

PARENTAL GPS

Parents and mentors don't need a map—just hearts brave enough to lead the way.

Raising a child isn't about following the perfect road map—it's about showing up with love and intention. We often think we need all the answers: the right schools, the right words, the right choices. But life teaches us otherwise. It humbles us. It shows us that presence matters more than perfection. Children don't need flawless parents, and people don't need infallible guides—they need present ones.

We can become careful chauffeurs of children's dreams, steering them through joy and heartbreak, failure and growth. Like any skilled driver, we adjust our course without panic. We trust our instincts when the path ahead is uncertain. We don't need to see every turn. We just need to stay beside them, consistently and lovingly.

Our children—our own and those entrusted to us—aren't asking for perfection; they're asking for presence. And when we lead with heart, the way forward always becomes clear.

Pause and reflect on the quiet power of parenting, mentoring, and shepherding. You're not just guiding schedules—you're guiding souls. Let your heart lead. Encourage their dreams, comfort their fears, and trust that your love is the most reliable compass they'll ever know.

How will you let your heart guide someone today?

APRIL 21

STOP CARRYING THE MOUNTAIN

Mountains are meant to be climbed, not carried.

Challenges ultimately aren't meant to weigh you down. They're meant to help you rise up. But often we mistake the mountain for a burden. We carry its weight in our mind, our body, and our spirit, dragging what was meant to be climbed.

The result? Exhaustion without elevation.

Mountains test you. They stretch you. They require strength, focus, and heart. But they're not meant to break you. They're meant to *build* you. When you climb, you grow. You learn where to place your next step. You pause when you need to. You rise, inch by inch, into a version of yourself you haven't yet met.

You don't have to carry the entire journey on your back. You just need to keep moving forward—one steady, intentional step at a time.

Put down the weight. Lace up your boots. Begin your ascent. The mountain has never been your burden to carry. The mountain holds your path to rise.

Are you carrying something you were meant to climb? How can you put it down and reach for the summit today?

THE KEY TO PERSPECTIVE

The door marked "obstacle" and the door marked "opportunity" open to the same room.

Two people can face the exact same challenge—yet each will walk away with a completely different outcome. Why? Because mind-set is the filter through which we experience reality. What appears to be a wall might actually be a doorway—if we're willing to see it that way. Perspective doesn't change what is happening, but it does change *what's possible* in the face of it. The situation doesn't hold the power. You do—when you assign meaning to what's in front of you.

Growth, strength, and transformation often wear the disguise of difficulty. The moment you shift from asking *Why is this happening to me?* to *What is this here to teach me?*, everything will begin to open up. The key is perspective—it may open doors you never knew existed.

When a challenge arises, choose to meet it with curiosity instead of resistance. Ask yourself: *What might this difficulty reveal? How could it serve me?* Adjust your lens, and what once felt like a burden may become your breakthrough.

What perspective shift could turn your next obstacle into an opportunity?

LETTING GO SO YOU CAN GROW

You will become who you're truly meant to be only when you let go of who you're not.

Becoming isn't about adding more. In fact, it's often about letting go. Many of us carry roles, labels, and expectations that we've outgrown or were never ours in the first place. We hold on to past mistakes, outdated identities, and versions of ourselves built more for survival than for joy.

These past versions may feel familiar and safe, but they can weigh us down and hold us back. Real transformation begins when we're brave enough to release our need to prove ourselves, to let go of perfection, to release the story that says we must be who we've always been.

When we shed these layers, something powerful happens. We begin to uncover the version of ourselves that's been waiting underneath all along. The truest becoming isn't about becoming more; it's about becoming *you*. Stronger. Lighter. Freer.

Ask yourself: *What roles, beliefs, or expectations am I holding on to that no longer reflect who I truly am? What am I willing to release so I can rise?* Growth doesn't necessarily mean adding. Real growth often begins with subtracting what no longer fits. Honor who you are becoming by courageously letting go.

What part of yourself are you ready to release so the real you can rise?

THE BRIDGE OF UNDERSTANDING

True understanding isn't built by speaking louder—it's built by listening deeper.

Sometimes, to be truly heard, we have to begin with what someone is *ready* to hear. Only then can we guide them toward what they need to understand. Real communication requires more than expressing ourselves clearly. We also must create connection. At times, we may feel the urge to offer insight, advice, or truth too soon, before the other person is open to receiving it. But experience teaches that timing and empathy matter just as much as the message itself.

Before we can lead someone across a bridge of understanding, we must first meet them where they are. When we start by listening—by acknowledging their feelings, their beliefs, their fears—we invite openness. And in that space of mutual respect, the conversation shifts from pushing ideas to exploring them together. That's where true connection and understanding happen.

Think of someone you're trying to reach right now. Rather than pushing your viewpoint, pause and reflect on theirs. Echo their emotions. Respect their pace. Then, gently offer your truth. You're not backing down from your message. You're prioritizing the connection first. Bridges aren't built by force. They're built by understanding.

Who in your life needs you to meet them where they are?

APRIL 25

THE ART OF REWIRING

Everyone has a loose wire now and then. What matters is noticing it without fear and patiently reconnecting it.

We've all had those days when something just feels "off"—a quiet disconnect we can't quite name. In those moments, we might feel the instinct to panic, push harder, or judge ourselves for not being fully "on." But moments like this aren't signs of failure—they're gentle invitations to pause.

Life shakes us sometimes. A stressful event, a tough conversation, or even subtle shifts like the shortening of days in winter can rattle our sense of balance. But like a skilled technician who doesn't panic over a loose wire, we too can meet these disruptions with steady awareness. These moments aren't breakdowns; they're signals, opportunities to realign. When we give ourselves space through rest, reflection, and presence, we begin to reconnect.

Rewiring isn't about fixing something that's broken. You're simply returning to what is real, what is true, and what is quietly waiting beneath the noise.

The next time you feel off-balance or emotionally frayed, resist the urge to judge the feeling or rush through it. Instead, ask yourself: *What part of me needs gentle attention right now?* Breathe, listen, and take one small step toward reconnection. You're not falling apart; you're being invited to reset.

What will you do today to gently reconnect with yourself?

YOU ARE THE ARCHITECT OF YOUR MIND

Consciousness doesn't ask us to silence our thoughts. It allows us to choose how we respond to them.

Our minds are always active. Thoughts rise and fall like waves. Some inspire us, others distract. The key to peace isn't in stopping our thoughts; it's in observing them without being consumed by them.

Consciousness means noticing what enters the mind and choosing how (or whether) to engage. Too often, we mistake mental noise for truth, reacting to every inner thought as if it defines us. But not every thought deserves a reaction or even our attention.

When we slow down and create space between thought and response, we tap into our greatest power: *awareness*. In that space, we learn to discern which thoughts build us up, which ones focus us, and which ones pull us off course. We become less reactive and more intentional. And in that shift, we transform from being ruled by our minds to designing how our minds work for us.

Take a moment to step back from your thoughts. Notice what's arising. Then ask: *Is this thought helpful? Is it aligned with who I want to be?* Write down your observations. Respond with clarity, not habit. You'll begin to shape your inner world with purpose, and that's where true freedom lives.

How will you use your awareness today to lead your thoughts rather than follow them?

ONE BREATH AT A TIME

When faced with a big task, stay grounded. Keep it simple—one step, one choice, one breath at a time.

Overwhelm has a way of distorting perspective—it makes the task ahead look like a mountain too steep to climb. But most accomplishments, no matter how massive, are achieved the same way—step by step. The greatest success comes from steady momentum and thoughtful progress, fueled by presence and intention.

When we focus on the next right move instead of on the entire journey, we give ourselves space to find clarity and regain our footing. Even in the face of uncertainty or intense pressure, it is always possible to take one breath, to make one small decision, to move one inch forward.

The moment we stop trying to conquer it all at once and instead ground ourselves in the present, we find power in steadiness.

If something in your life feels overwhelming, take a pause. Breathe. Ask yourself: *What one small thing can I do right now to relieve some of the pressure?* Clarity and answers will come as you ground yourself in simplicity and presence.

What would change if you stopped chasing the finish line and instead focused on the next step?

THE TIMING OF WISDOM

Wisdom is knowing when to pause and when to act, moving in step with opportunity.

One of the most overlooked truths is that doing the right thing at the wrong time can still lead to the wrong outcome. We've all rushed forward, mistaking urgency for momentum, only to force open doors that weren't meant to be opened. And we've all waited far too long for something, paralyzed by fear or doubt, only to watch opportunities quietly pass us by.

Wisdom isn't just about knowing what the next step is. It's about recognizing *when to take it*. Life moves at a rhythm, and when we learn to listen to that beat, our choices will align with something deeper than pressure or fear. When our actions are in sync with that rhythm, they are smoother, more powerful, and more meaningful.

Timing isn't about speed. It's about alignment. When we act from intention instead of impulse, true momentum will follow.

Take a moment today to reflect: *Am I pushing when I should be waiting? Or am I waiting when it's time to move?* Turn inward. Listen. Let patience and courage guide you when the moment calls.

What opportunity in your life is asking for patience? What is asking for bold, timely action?

THE MEASURE OF TRUE SUCCESS

True success is measured not by what you achieve but by the lives you touch along the way.

We often chase milestones, recognition, and results, believing that success is measured in accolades. But the deeper truth is that trophies gather dust, titles fade, and accomplishments gradually lose some of their meaning.

What endures is *impact*. The lives you touch. The voices you encourage. The strength you lend to others when they're too tired to stand. True success isn't about reaching the top alone—it's about reaching back a hand to bring others along on the ascent. Success is found in the quiet moments when your words soften someone's fear or your presence becomes another person's hope. It's the compassion woven into your ambition and the service embedded in your achievements.

When your journey becomes a source of light for someone else's path, your legacy truly begins. Success that serves only the self may shine briefly, but success that uplifts others becomes timeless.

Ask yourself: *In my pursuit of success, who am I bringing with me?* Use your strengths not just to build your own success but to elevate those around you. Let your wins open doors for others. The highest form of success isn't in measuring who's standing tallest but in rising together.

What part of your journey can become someone else's inspiration today?

THE POWER OF CALMNESS

In the middle of conflict, your power lies in your calmness, not your desire to control.

In the heat of conflict, it's easy to believe that the loudest voice will win. But true power isn't found in volume or control—it's found in presence. Calmness doesn't mean passivity. Calmness signals that a person is grounded. Steady energy keeps you rooted when emotions run high.

When you listen with genuine intent—not just to respond, but to understand—you defuse tension instead of stoking it. When you lead with respect, you invite the same in return. Conflict doesn't have to be a battlefield. It can be a bridge. The goal isn't to overpower—it's to find resolution that honors both truth and connection. You can be firm without being forceful. You can stand your ground without stepping on someone else's toes. There's a compelling power in calmness.

When conflict arises, choose calmness. Take a breath before you speak. Aim to understand, not to win. Lead the way toward resolution—not through force, but through focused presence and respect.

When tension rises, do you reach for control or do you return to calm?

MAY

MAY 1

SPARKS OF CONNECTION

Human connection isn't just comfort—
it's the fuel for hope and optimism.

Even the strongest among us needs connection. Connection isn't a luxury. It's a lifeline, our deepest purpose during our time on earth. In moments of doubt, exhaustion, or loneliness, isolation isn't what restores confidence or revives the spirit. It's human connection that pulls us back from the brink, lifts us out of sadness, and brings joy to a broken heart.

A kind word. A gentle touch. A conversation in which we feel truly seen. These small moments carry the power to restore what we may have thought was lost. Healing begins with connection. Relationship renews our strength and gives hope footing.

It's easy to believe we must carry the burdens of life alone, but we are wired to belong, to be supported, and to support in return. Another's simple presence, listening and caring, is enough to breathe life back into the places that had gone cold.

Don't wait for the "right time" to connect. Reach out. Call a friend, look someone in the eye, ask a deeper question. Give another person your full attention. Be the one who listens without judgment. These sparks of connection will light the way forward.

Who in your life needs a spark of connection today, and are you willing to offer it?

CHOOSE CALM AMID CHAOS

True power is choosing calm when chaos calls.

Anger can surge in us like a tidal wave—sudden, intense, capable of crushing everything in its path. In those moments, it may feel freeing and even powerful to lash out, to react, to assert control through force. But the ramifications of doing so are costly.

Often, anger is rooted in the fear of losing something important to us, whether that's respect, safety, love, or control. But we won't find power in the outburst. True power waits in the pause of a steadying breath. Mastering our emotional responses doesn't mean denying what we feel. Instead, we must work to understand the emotion, own it, and recognize the deeper fear beneath it.

When we choose to respond thoughtfully rather than react, we open the door to clarity, empathy, and intentional action. Real transformation happens when we choose calm over chaos.

The next time chaos comes knocking—whether in a conversation, a challenge, or your own thoughts—pause. Ground yourself. Ask: *Is this the moment when I roar . . . or the moment when I reset?* Choose stillness over reaction. That decision, made consistently, will build the kind of strength that leads, heals, and inspires.

What will you do the next time the storm surges inside you?

THE POWER OF "NO"

"No" isn't rejection; it's a boundary. It's not a harsh word, just a clear answer that's meant to be respected.

Many of us are ingrained with the belief that saying no is selfish or unkind. We equate being agreeable and available with being good. But every time we say yes when we mean no, we trade honesty for approval—and lose a little of our peace in the process.

The truth is, "no" isn't a rejection. It's an act of self-respect. Boundaries aren't barriers; they're foundations for healthier, more authentic relationships. When we say no, we prevent resentment from festering. We create space for honesty instead of silent frustration. By honoring our limits, we allow others to trust our yes even more. Saying no isn't about closing doors. It's about opening the right ones with clarity, confidence, and care—and protecting your energy in the process.

Today, give yourself permission to say no. If a request, invitation, or obligation doesn't align with your values or capacity, it's okay to decline. Practice saying no with kindness and conviction. Remember: Your energy is a resource, not an obligation. When you honor your boundaries, you teach others how to respect them too.

Where in your life do you need to say no so you can say yes to yourself?

THE SPACE BETWEEN HOPE AND FEAR

Hope and fear cannot share the same space. One will always emerge as the other fades into the distance.

Inside each of us lives a powerful pull—between fear and hope. Fear is quick to take hold. And when it does, it clouds your thinking, weighs down your spirit, and makes even the smallest step feel impossible. But hope—quiet, steady, and persistent—waits for you to reach out and choose it. And when you do, fear begins to loosen its grip, clarity returns, and new possibilities open before you.

Hope isn't blind optimism. It's the belief that no matter how uncertain things may seem, something better is possible. Hope doesn't deny fear's existence. It simply refuses to let fear lead. The more you choose hope, the more resilient you become. Hope brings light to dark places, strength to weary hearts, and courage when you're ready to give up.

You can't nurture both fear and hope. Choose to nurture the one that lifts you.

Are you feeding fear or allowing hope to grow? Invite hope in, even if only in a whisper. Let it guide your next step, your next breath, your next decision. When hope leads, your life will begin to align with possibility.

What would shift if, instead of letting fear close doors, you allowed hope to open them?

MAY 5

GROWTH HURTS BEFORE IT HEALS

No one builds strength—physical or emotional—without some discomfort.

The most meaningful breakthroughs rarely arrive wrapped in comfort or ease. Whether it's the physical strain of a workout, the emotional tension of honest conversations, or the inner pull of self-reflection, growth almost always comes with challenge. Often the hardest part is beginning—because we sense how much it might hurt. We doubt the reward could outweigh the struggle, but it always does.

Discomfort isn't the enemy. It's a signal. It means you're pushing past what's familiar, expanding into something new. Just like muscles strengthen through resistance, our minds and hearts grow stronger when we're stretched beyond our usual limits. The key isn't to avoid the discomfort but to recognize it for what it is: proof that transformation is underway. The stretch may be uncomfortable, but it's temporary. The rewarding growth that follows? That's what lasts—and heals us.

In what areas of your life are you avoiding discomfort? What have you been hesitant to face because of the pain that might come with it? Lean into it. The next time you feel the strain, whether in your body or in your spirit, look at it as evidence that you're changing and getting stronger.

What discomfort are you willing to embrace today for the sake of who you're becoming?

THE MEANING OF LONGEVITY

Longevity isn't defined by a number of years—it's the depth, direction, and dedication put into those years.

For much of our lives, we're taught to see longevity as the goal—to live longer, stay active, defy the passage of time. Culture today glorifies youth and often acts like aging is some kind of failure, but many of us have begun to realize that a greater number of years means very little if those years don't have meaning. A life stretched for many miles but lacking purpose can feel hollow, while a brief life filled with presence and purpose seems infinite.

True longevity isn't measured in distance but in depth. It's about living with intention, aligning your actions with your values, and nurturing the practices—mental, physical, emotional, and spiritual—that sustain you. Longevity is about more than adding days to your life. True longevity is adding life to your days.

Pause and ask yourself: *Am I merely counting the days, or am I making the days count?* Longevity takes on deeper meaning when you stop focusing on time and instead invest in depth of experience, clarity of purpose, and consistency in self-care. Let each moment be a conscious investment in a life that feels truly *alive*.

What one intentional change can you make today to live more deeply instead of just trying to live longer?

LOOK DEEPER

Behind every face are oceans of untold stories. Judge softly. You see only the surface, not the depths below.

It's easy to judge what you can see—a reaction, a habit, a moment in time. But what you're seeing is just the surface. Beneath every external behavior you witness is a depth you can't see and haven't lived: private struggles, silent victories, invisible wounds, resilient hopes. The loudest person might be carrying loneliness. The quietest one might be shouldering mountains.

When you rush to label, you miss the chance to understand. You see only the ripple and miss the ocean. But when you pause and lead with empathy, you make space for connection instead of assumption. You don't have to know the depths of a person's story to choose kindness. Just remember there *is* a story—and you're only catching a glimpse.

You wouldn't judge the ocean by a single wave. Don't judge a person by a single moment.

The next time you're tempted to judge, slow down. Get curious. Offer grace. Let your presence be a safe space, not a spotlight. More is happening beneath the surface than you'll ever know.

Where in your life could deeper understanding replace quick judgment? What would that shift open up for you?

LETTING LOVE LEAD

Is love speaking? Or is wounded pride, hiding behind the need to be right, dominating your interactions?

In life's toughest conversations, sometimes our words are motivated by love—balanced, calm, and rooted in connection. At other times, our words are being guided by pride disguised as logic or self-protection.

We've all said things just to feel right, to "win," or to avoid vulnerability. We've defended positions we knew weren't true because to admit being wrong would leave us too exposed. And every time pride takes the lead, it costs us—moments of closeness, opportunities for healing, and chances to understand and be understood.

But when we let love shape our words, even difficult truths can land with grace. Leading with love doesn't mean weakness or surrender. It means choosing our tone with intention, gauging our timing with care, and seasoning our words with compassion. It's not about being right—it's about being real and choosing connection over control.

In the heat of a conflict, stop and ask yourself: *What part of me is doing the talking? What is steering my thoughts before I even speak?* Before you say a word, commit to connecting with the part of you that is rooted in love and choose words that unite.

What would shift in your relationships if you let love take the lead in your communication?

MAY 9

THE HIDDEN WORLD

Where do people vanish to when they step into the online realm?

A strange phenomenon is happening in our world. We're in the room, but we're not really there. We're surrounded by others, yet we're scrolling through some other place—eyes fixed on a screen, mind drifting, connections fading as we fall deeper into the scroll.

We've all reached for our phone instead of staying present in the moment, numbing discomfort rather than facing it. While the digital world offers entertainment, knowledge, and connection, it also offers an escape from the here and now. This escape isn't inherently wrong, but when it becomes a reflex, a default, you risk losing touch with what's real: the people around you, the energy in the room, the peace found in stillness.

Choose to be mindful as you engage with social media. Let technology serve you rather than steal from you. What truly matters isn't on a screen—it's the people around you. And those people are hoping you'll look up.

Before your next scroll, ask yourself: *Am I escaping or engaging?* Stay grounded in the here and now. Use technology to support your growth, but don't allow it to replace your reality.

How can you create more intentional space in your day to disconnect from devices and reconnect with what—and who—matters most?

THE PRISON OR THE PORTAL

The mind can be a prison or a portal—you can either be trapped inside or observe from the outside.

The mind holds incredible power. It can limit us or liberate us depending on how we engage with it. When thoughts are left unchecked—especially those rooted in fear, doubt, or judgment—they can shackle us, creating an illusion of limitation.

But there's another way. When we step back and observe our thoughts with awareness instead of attachment, something shifts. That act of witnessing turns the mind from a cage to a compass. We begin to see patterns, gain perspective, and uncover insights that were buried beneath noise.

You don't have to silence your thoughts or pretend they don't exist. You have the power to choose not to be consumed by them. And in that choice, you access the portal to clarity, creativity, and transformation.

Take a moment today to tune in. Notice your thoughts, especially the ones that tend to spiral. Rather than reacting, pause and ask yourself: *Is this thought helping me or holding me back?* Through that one simple question, you can reclaim your power. The mind isn't a trap. It can be your guide . . . if you learn to see it clearly.

What thought or story have you been trapped inside? How might observing it shift your path?

PUSHING BEYOND LIMITS

When you feel you can't go any further, take just one more step—however small.

We've all met our limits—during tough workouts, exhausting days, or creative blocks when nothing seems to flow. In those moments, it's easy to believe we have nothing left. Muscles shake. Doubt creeps in. The mind says, "That's enough."

But something powerful happens when we go just a *little* further—that final rep, that last task, that trip back to the creative well. Those moments reveal strength we might not realize we have. What we often think of as limits are actually thresholds we haven't crossed yet.

When you lean in, especially when everything inside says to stop, you don't just push past the roadblock; you also grow. Each time you stretch beyond what you thought was possible, you redefine your edge—and prove to yourself you're capable of more than you imagined.

Whatever challenge you're facing right now—mental, physical, emotional—know that you have more in you. When you hit a wall, take a breath and then take one more step, however big or small. Perseverance doesn't ask you to leap. Just lean forward, take it one step at a time, and you'll go further than you believed possible.

What might you discover about yourself if you pushed beyond your limits?

THE POWER OF PERSISTENCE

Persistence reminds us that with every step forward, no matter how small, we're one step closer to our goal.

Persistence isn't always loud. It's not the victory lap or the cheers from the crowd. Persistence is that quiet decision to keep going, especially when the finish line feels far away. It's in the days when motivation is missing, but you show up anyway. When results are invisible, but your effort doesn't waver.

Progress isn't always a sudden breakthrough. It's built in repetition, in small wins, in the courage to begin again when you fall. Each small act of consistency—one breath, one rep, one honest step—strengthens your path and reshapes your future. You may not feel the change right away, but persistence lays the groundwork for transformation.

What you do regularly—however small—will always matter more than what you do occasionally. So don't confuse slow with stuck. You're not failing. You're steadily forging a foundation that will not fail you.

Take one step today—just one—that honors your goal. Write one line. Do one set of stretches. Make one bold decision. Then choose to take another step tomorrow. That's persistence. That's progress. And that's how lasting success is built.

Where in your life could one small act today create the momentum your future self has been waiting for?

POWER *IS* SERVICE

Power doesn't come from putting others down. Real power lifts others up.

True power isn't demonstrated through dominance, control, or pride. It's revealed in humility—in the quiet moments when you use your voice, your presence, or your influence to benefit others. The most powerful people aren't always the loudest or the center of attention. Often those making the *most* difference, enacting the *most* change, are the ones who listen deeply, lead with empathy, and elevate others without demanding the spotlight.

Perhaps you once believed that being powerful meant hiding your struggles, never showing vulnerability, or always seeking recognition. But real power is being secure enough to help someone else shine—even if it means stepping back and letting them take the spotlight.

Power built on ego will eventually collapse. But power rooted in compassion is unshakable.

Take a moment today to reflect: *Am I using my power to uplift others or to overshadow them?* The world doesn't need more people fighting to be the tallest, the most respected, the most powerful. The world needs people who are willing to be humble, reach out, and lift up. Use your power to support others, not as a superiority tactic.

What would our world look like if every act of power was also an act of service?

POWER IN ALIGNMENT

We thrive when body, mind, heart, and spirit align—all parts moving as one.

You aren't one dimensional. You are a symphony of the physical, mental, emotional, and spiritual. And when just one part falls out of rhythm or out of tune, the entire melody shifts. You can't meditate your way through burnout while ignoring your body's cries for rest. You can't push for progress if your spirit feels lost or your heart is shut down.

True power isn't achieved by domination in one area of life. We step into it through integration—when body, mind, heart, and spirit move together. When the body is nourished, the mind clears. When the heart is open, actions find purpose. When the spirit is grounded, one's whole being knows its direction. Alignment doesn't demand perfection. It simply asks for presence, thoughtfulness, and intentional action in each part of who you are.

Take a moment today to check in with each part of yourself. Are you ignoring your needs? Are you pushing one part while silencing another? Move your body with intention. Sit in quiet to hear your truth. Lead with both strength and softness. When all of you shows up in harmony, you rise into your power.

What part of you may have been left unheard? How can you bring it back into alignment today?

THE VALUE OF TRUE CONNECTION

Seek out the deep love and understanding of a true friend.

The applause of the crowd can be intoxicating, but it's only temporary. That type of praise rises with your wins and fades just as quickly when the spotlight moves on. What remains steady is the quiet loyalty of someone who truly knows you—someone who celebrates you, not for your image but for your essence, someone who sees your flaws and stays anyway.

Applause may feed the ego, but real connection nourishes the soul. In a world obsessed with followers, likes, and endless attention, it's easy to forget what—or *who*—matters most: the few who genuinely listen, care, and stand beside you when there's no audience around. Love from those steady, constant friends who truly know you is transformative. A single honest connection can hold more healing than a thousand cheers.

Nurture the relationships that truly matter—the ones that bring depth, not just attention. In a world obsessed with appearances, choose substance. Reach out to someone who's always had your back, and remind them they're seen, valued, and loved.

Who in your life offers genuine connection? How can you strengthen that bond today?

STEER YOUR SHIP

The direction you choose, not the distance, will shape your journey the most.

How fast you move or how far you go doesn't define your journey. The direction in which you point your ship is what matters. We all have times when we move quickly, check boxes, and make progress, only to realize we're heading away from what truly matters. We also have seasons where progress feels slow or even invisible and yet every step is intentional, aligned, and on course.

True growth isn't measured by distance but by purpose. If your path is taking you further from your values or your truth, distance means very little. The moment you choose a direction that reflects who you are and what you stand for—and then choose actions that keep you on course—is when your journey truly begins.

Even the smallest shift in course, made with clarity, can lead to the greatest change in direction.

Today, ask yourself: *Am I headed in the direction that aligns with who I want to become?* If not, be ready to pivot. One small shift now can completely redefine your destination. Making sure you're going in the right direction matters far more than the speed with which you get there.

What small course correction can you make today to move closer to your true destination?

STRENGTH IN UNITY

Relationships aren't a competition—lift each other up, inspire growth, and succeed together.

The strongest relationships aren't built on rivalry—they're built on mutual respect, trust, and support. When you stop measuring who's ahead and start focusing on how you can rise together, everything shifts.

True unity happens when success becomes shared, not compared. You grow faster when you celebrate each other's wins and see each other's growth as inspiration instead of a threat. You shine brighter together when you create space for each other's light. Support doesn't weaken your path—it strengthens your character. It builds a foundation of safety where both people can evolve. In a world that often pushes you to compete, choosing connection over comparison becomes a powerful act of emotional maturity and love. Real partnerships—romantic, personal, and professional—aren't about who leads. They're about how far you can go together.

Examine your relationships. Are you subtly competing with others or actively supporting them? Set the scoreboard aside. Be a source of strength, not pressure. Celebrate the wins that aren't yours. Be a mirror for someone else's greatness. Real success isn't about being first. It's about rising—side by side.

How might your relationships change if you chose collaboration over comparison?

REDIRECTION, NOT REJECTION

Rejection is life guiding you toward
the people and places who won't just
tolerate your light, but celebrate it.

It stings to be excluded. Whether it's silence, a closed door, or being overlooked, rejection feels personal. But what if it's not a verdict—what if it's a nudge? A quiet, forceful redirection toward something better aligned, more life-giving, more *you*?

Not everyone or everything is meant for you—and that's a gift.

Every "no" saves you from chasing what's misaligned. It clears space for what's real. For what doesn't just accept you—but calls you to your higher purpose and truest self.

Rejection is often protection in disguise. A sacred reroute away from environments that stifle and toward spaces that empower. When you're brave enough to keep walking, you eventually find your people in those who reflect your worth instead of questioning it.

Release the need to be chosen by those who can't see you, and make room for those who do. Find the people and spaces that greet your light with mirrors instead of shades. Your light was never meant to be hidden.

Where have you mistaken rejection for failure—and how might it actually be life pushing you toward something more authentic?

ADDICTED TO BUSYNESS

Constant activity can become an elegant addiction, drowning out the silence we're afraid to listen to.

Busyness may feel productive, but constant motion is often a clever disguise. We fill our schedules, check off tasks, and chase achievements not necessarily because they matter but because they keep us distracted.

There's nothing inherently wrong with productivity. It can be fulfilling and even beautiful. But when it becomes a way to avoid reality, to shy away from discomfort or procrastinate genuine transformation, productivity is no longer serving us but is instead shielding us—from the truths we fear, the discomfort we resist, and the selves we're meant to become.

In those rare quiet moments we so often resist, truth, clarity, and healing have space to rise. Stillness reveals what speed conceals: unmet needs, quiet desires, the redirection we've been avoiding. Action has power, but it first must be rooted in purpose. Without that, it's simply noise. The world will always celebrate your hustle, but only you can give your stillness the respect it deserves.

Take a break today—not because you're burned out but because you're brave enough to listen. Let the silence speak. Let it reveal what the noise has drowned out.

What might you discover if you stopped being busy long enough to truly feel?

TRUE WEALTH

True wealth isn't the size of your bank account. It's measured in freedom, harmony, and purpose.

True wealth isn't defined by a number. It's measured by how deeply we connect, align, and find peace. Some people with great financial success feel empty, chasing the next big purchase or status symbol but never reaching wholeness. Others find richness in life's simplest moments—time spent in nature, laughter with loved ones, living with purpose.

Wealth, in its most meaningful form, is the freedom to be who you are without apology. It's the inner harmony that comes from being in balance and the clarity that comes from knowing why you're here. When those pieces fall into place, life feels full—no matter how much is in your bank account.

Real abundance comes from within. And when we measure wealth by depth of experience and relationship rather than in dollars, we'll realize we've had more than enough all along.

Ask yourself today: *What kind of wealth am I really building?* Are you focused solely on income, or are you also investing in your well-being, your relationships, your sense of meaning? Begin to redirect your energy toward the things that make life feel whole. Real wealth isn't something you hold on to; it's something you live.

What can you start nurturing today to create a richer, fuller life?

"LATER" IS A LIE

Procrastination is the enemy of change. What is postponed for later is often never done at all.

I'll do it later." We've all said it—but "later" is a lie. It lulls us into comfort, making us believe we can pretend that postponing progress is just a pause as we wait for the right moment. But what we push aside often stays there, discarded and forgotten.

Procrastination isn't laziness. It's often fear in disguise. Fear of failure. Fear of discomfort. Fear of what growth might demand of us. But every time we delay, we reinforce the false belief that now isn't the right time. That belief becomes habit, and habit becomes our identity.

If you're waiting for the perfect moment, here it is—the perfect moment is *now*. Not tomorrow. Not next week. Start immediately, and momentum will do the rest. The sooner you begin, the sooner you'll move through the discomfort and into the transformation waiting on the other side.

Whatever it is you've been putting off, take the first small step today. Don't wait for confidence. Let movement create confidence. Stop treating "later" like a promise.

What decision or action have you been postponing that would bring change if you started addressing it today?

THE WEIGHT OF WORDS

Words have the power to build or destroy. Choose them wisely.

Words are more than sounds. Words are *seeds*. Once spoken, they land somewhere: in hearts, in minds, in memories. And like seeds, they grow. They can become shelter like the branches of a vast tree . . . or they can take root as weeds, forcing their way in and leaving behind scars. A careless word can wound in ways that even time struggles to heal. But a sincere phrase of encouragement, empathy, or love can release positive echoes for a lifetime.

That's the unseen power we carry every time we speak. We often underestimate how much of our world is built from language. How we speak to others shapes our relationships. How we talk to ourselves shapes our identity. If you want to speak with intention, you must live with awareness. Be conscious of what comes out of your mouth, and honor the fact that your words can plant fields of abundance wherever you go.

Pause before you speak today. Ask yourself: *Will these words uplift or diminish? Clarify or confuse? Heal or harden?* Once released, words don't vaporize. They *take root*. Let your language become a force for good.

Think of a moment when someone's words changed you. Was it for better or for worse?

MAY 23

PEACE IN THE PRESENT

Anxiety arises from borrowing tomorrow's troubles for today. Peace lives in the present.

Peace isn't achieved once we've solved every problem or predicted future challenges and planned for every possible outcome. Peace is available when we slow down enough to notice what is happening *now*, when we're present in this exact moment. Anxiety often thrives in future thinking, feeding off stories we haven't yet lived and outcomes we can't control. The present, by contrast, is simpler. It's quieter. And it's where peace lives.

When you stop forecasting and worrying and instead focus on the moment at hand—your breath, your senses, your surroundings—you create space between yourself and the storm in your mind. And in that space, peace is waiting to meet you. Yes, the future matters. But you can't address the future *right now.* You meet the future one moment at a time by staying present, grounded, and aware.

The present isn't the enemy of progress; it's the foundation on which progress is built.

When anxiety strikes, bring yourself back to the present. Breathe. Name five things you see. Feel your feet on the ground. Remind yourself: *This moment is manageable.* You can face tomorrow—but only by standing fully in today.

What one thing can you do right now to anchor yourself in the present and reclaim your peace?

STRENGTH IN ADAPTATION

People and circumstances are ever-changing—
wisdom lies in our ability to adapt.

Life is constantly shifting beneath our feet—unexpected financial issues, illness, stress at work, relationships that need tending. In my experience, the more we try to control life, the more it resists our grip. If we cling to how things were *supposed to be*, we may end up missing what they *could be*.

You've likely been there—navigating altered plans, unexpected U-turns, shifting roles. Life is constantly in motion, and real growth comes when we learn to move with intention through the slalom course of life. The ability to adapt reveals a quiet strength, the skill to accept and then adjust course. You're strong enough to bend without breaking, grounded enough to plot a new course, and wise enough to let go of the old to make space for what's next.

Ask yourself: *Where am I resisting the natural flow of life? What am I afraid to release, even if it no longer serves me?* Choose one area where you can let go of control and lean into curiosity. Adapting doesn't mean you're abandoning your path; you're simply adjusting your stride.

What part of you is ready to stop resisting and start adapting?

TAKE OFF THE MASK

If you want to be seen for who you truly are,
put down the masks you hide behind.

As we journey through life, we put on various masks crafted from expectations, fear, and the desire to belong. We present curated versions of ourselves to escape judgment, rejection, or vulnerability. Perhaps it's a mask of false confidence. Or maybe you only allow people to see the version of you who never has a bad day. But with each mask we don, we grow more distant from our truth. Masks may earn us approval, but they don't bring peace—because what others are accepting isn't the complete *you.*

Authenticity doesn't mean you have to broadcast every detail of your life. You still own your story. Authenticity means honoring what's real and having the courage to speak your truth, even if your voice trembles. It's choosing to be seen rather than admired.

When you stop performing, you will begin connecting. And when you let go of who you think you *should* be, you will finally embrace who you *are.*

Take one small step toward authenticity today. Say what you mean. Share what you feel. Let someone see behind the mask. That's where freedom, strength, and true belonging begin.

What part of your authentic self is ready to be seen today? How can you let it shine?

THE TRANSFORMATIVE QUESTION

What's holding you back from the life you were meant to live?

What's holding you back? It's a question that cuts to the core. At first, your answers might sound logical: lack of time, support, or opportunity. But when we look deeper, the real answers to what is holding us back often point inward.

Behind the delay is fear.

Behind the hesitation is doubt.

The safety of the known keeps us small.

The weight of an old story that once protected you now limits your future.

The truth is, most walls aren't built outside us—they're built within. But the moment you name what's really in the way, what's really holding you back, you reclaim the power to push through it. You don't need to dismantle the entire wall at once. Awareness will create an opening. And from that crack your courage will grow.

Find a quiet moment and ask: *What's really holding me back?* Don't overthink it. Just listen. Be honest and kind to yourself. Then ask a second question: *What small step can I take today to move forward?* That step, however slight, holds the power to change everything.

Are you ready to stop waiting and start becoming who you were always meant to be?

CHOOSE YOU

Choose peace over chaos. Choose clarity over noise. Most of all, choose you.

Every day we're offered choices. They're not always big, dramatic choices. Some are quiet and constant: the choice to react or respond, to absorb noise or protect clarity, to chase approval or return to the self.

These daily and repeated decisions shape the rhythm of our lives more than any single event ever could. Peace isn't always the easiest choice—it requires letting go of what's loud, toxic, or familiar. Clarity doesn't scream for attention. It whispers beneath the surface, waiting for you to drown out the rest of the noise and listen. And choosing *you*? That's the boldest move of all. It means honoring your boundaries, trusting your voice, and believing that your well-being matters—not someday but *now*.

You don't owe the world your burnout. You owe it your truth. And that truth will emerge when you choose yourself again and again, without guilt.

> Pause and ask yourself: *Is this choice or action bringing me peace or pulling me into chaos?* Make your next move a conscious one, and choose yourself.

Where in your life are you ready to choose yourself—and what will that look like starting now?

RETURN TO THE BEGINNING

When you hit a dead end, return to where it all began to find clarity and forge a new path.

Sometimes when we feel lost or off course, we force our way forward. We keep pushing, as if forward motion equals progress.

Instead of forcing whatever it is, pause and return to your origin. Revisit why you began whatever this pursuit is, what lit that first spark, and who you were before the noise muddied your focus. Clarity often comes when we stop pushing mindlessly and instead remember what mattered most in the first place.

Your deepest motivations—the ones rooted in passion and purpose—are still here, waiting to guide you back to alignment. You don't need to reinvent yourself or this dream. Sometimes all it takes is coming home to your truth so you can see the next step clearly. What once felt like a dead end becomes a turning point when you approach it with awareness and intention.

Go back to the beginning. What is your *why*? Write it down. The answers you've been seeking might not be ahead of you—they might actually be behind you, ready to light your path forward. Let that original fire guide your next move.

What belief did you once hold so strongly that it propelled you forward? How can you return to it now?

THE PRICE OF DECEIT

The merchant of deceit spares no one, for his gain is measured in the trust he betrays.

Deceit may offer the illusion of an easy path, promising that you'll avoid discomfort, secure an advantage, or bend reality in your favor. But every dishonest word or manipulated truth plants a seed of destruction, not just in the relationships it affects but in the soul of the person who speaks the lie.

Trust is more than just a bond; it's a sacred currency. And when trust has been recklessly spent through deception, what has been lost is rarely regained. The deceiver may walk away with what they want in the moment, but they leave behind a trail of doubt, disillusionment, and broken connection. Over time, their world will grow smaller, colder, lonelier. A life built on shadows, no matter how clever, will never know real connection.

True character is seen in how bravely you stand in truth. Honesty won't always be easy, but it will always pay off—in legacy, respect, and peace.

Be a steward of truth, not a merchant of manipulation. Choose honesty even when silence tempts you, even when deceit seems like an easier way out. The trust you preserve today becomes the foundation you stand on tomorrow.

What kind of foundation are you building with your words?

THE ARMOR OF OVERACHIEVING

Overworking isn't strength; it's an old wound disguised as worth.

Our culture glorifies "hustle." It equates doing more with being more, and burnout is often seen as dedication. But beneath that drive, what if ambition isn't what's pushing us? What if staying busy and overachieving are actually attempts at self-protection?

Giving too much—at work, in relationships—can become armor we put on to shield ourselves from the fear of inadequacy. We chase praise, productivity, and perfection, hoping they'll make us feel *enough*. But no amount of striving or success can heal whatever has made you feel unworthy. Healing can come only from allowing yourself to pause, to rest, to be cared for, and to acknowledge your inherent worth.

Reclaiming peace and worth begins when you separate your identity from productivity. You have *always* been enough, before the effort, before the success. And you will remain enough long after all the praise fades away.

Ask yourself: *Is this effort rooted in purpose or in fear?* If you realize you're operating out of fear of being less than, allow yourself to soften. You don't need to prove anything to be worthy of rest, love, or belonging. Be present with yourself and know your worth.

How might your life change if you stopped trying to prove your worth?

CHOOSE WHAT LASTS

Choose what lasts. Your peace is worth more than a moment's thrill.

Temptation doesn't always come in grand form. It can show up as a quick fix, a distraction, or a fleeting delight that promises relief in the moment. But not everything that feels good *is* good—especially if it costs you your peace. Maybe it's giving in to unfaithfulness, knowing the fallout will wound more than just yourself. Maybe it's letting someone stumble when you had the chance to lift them up. Or maybe it's saying yes to a "harmless" escape that only leaves you emptier when it's over. These choices may feel small, but they leave a weight that lingers long after the moment has passed.

Peace isn't just a nice benefit. Peace is your compass. It keeps you steady when the world tries to pull you in every direction. When you sacrifice your peace for temporary highs, you disconnect from your center.

The next time you're at a crossroads, ask yourself: *Will this thing serve me after the moment fades?* And then choose what lasts and what will feed your peace.

Protect your peace. Choose what will still feel right tomorrow, not just what feels good right now.

What would it look like to make decisions not just for this moment but for who you want to be tomorrow?

JUNE

WHEREVER YOU GO, THERE YOU ARE

Changing your address won't change your struggles. They simply unpack alongside you.

It's tempting to think that a fresh environment will fix whatever troubles us—that new surroundings will erase old pain. We're all familiar with this mind-set. *If I could just leave this job . . . this relationship . . . this town behind, everything would be better.*

Changing your environment *can* be powerful—and sometimes it's necessary for growth. A fresh start can breathe new life into your journey. But wherever you go, your inner world follows. The same doubts, fears, and patterns can reappear in different clothes, different cities, and different relationships.

True growth comes from facing what's inside. When we choose to do the inner work—to examine our patterns, heal old hurts, and take ownership of our mind-set—we create the kind of acceptance and peace that no relocation can deliver. And with that peace, we're able to stop running and start arriving—fully and wholly—wherever we are.

Before you chase a change of scenery, ask yourself: *What am I* really *trying to leave behind?* Sit with whatever that is. Once you confront your pain or mistakes and find peace within, you may realize you're already home.

What are you carrying that keeps following you? Arc you ready to face it before you move again?

THE TRUE VALUE OF GOOD DEEDS

The significance of a good deed isn't measured by the recognition it earns but by the heart it's born from.

It's natural to want our good deeds to be seen. It's entirely human to enjoy the feeling of another person noticing that you extended generosity, helped someone else, or donated your time or money.

Recognition feels good, but the most authentic form of giving doesn't seek an audience. True generosity aligns with your values. Pure kindness isn't performative or waiting for applause. Authentic giving shows up when no one's looking. It acts without needing credit. And in a world that often rewards image over intention, choosing quiet generosity becomes a radical act.

The most powerful gestures—the ones that stay with people—are often unseen. When your actions come from a place of sincerity, they carry a different kind of weight that can't be measured in likes or praise but in the quiet ripple effect of impacting another life.

The next time you offer help, encouragement, or kindness, pause and ask yourself: *Am I doing this for visibility and acknowledgment, or because of my values?* Let the action itself be the reward. Let your integrity guide your generosity.

What would your kindness look like if you stopped needing it to be seen?

THE QUIET POWER OF THE PAUSE

The best choices come from clarity and freedom, not from pressure or fear.

In a world that glorifies instant decisions and swift action, we often forget the quiet power of the pause. Fear can disguise itself as urgency, whispering that time is running out, that if we don't act now, we'll lose something vital.

But decisions made in haste rarely serve us. They come from reaction rather than from wisdom. Our ability to stop, breathe, and discern gives us power. We're not ignoring fear but instead refusing to be ruled by it. That intentional pause gives us the opportunity to find alignment—when we check in with our values, weigh our intentions, and step into conscious choice. The pause is where we remember who we are *beneath* the noise—where vision becomes clearer and pressure begins to fade.

We find freedom when we stop rushing in an attempt to avoid discomfort and instead trust ourselves enough to slow down, reflect, and respond with clarity and courage.

When urgency rises up inside you, instead of taking an immediate leap into action, take a breath. Ask yourself: *Is this coming from fear or from alignment?* Let your next move come from stillness rather than stress.

What would shift in your life if you honored the pause before every important decision?

THE SPACE TO BECOME

Growth doesn't rush. Growth unfolds when we make space for it.

Becoming who we're meant to be isn't about piling on more—additional obligations, loftier goals, higher expectations.

Becoming requires clearing space to breathe, to feel, to listen inward. Those quiet moments, away from the noise, away from voices and influences and perceived expectations, are when we're able to recognize more clearly what fuels us and what drains us.

Typically, it's not too hard to recognize what needs to go. The challenge tends to lie in finding the courage to release it. Whether it's an old belief, a draining routine, or simply too much of everything, letting go creates room—and time—for what matters most. What we choose to nurture—our values, our joy, our connections—shapes the life we're building. When you give yourself space to reflect on what to nurture and what to release, you will uncover the truth of who you are and who you're meant to become.

Find ten quiet minutes today. During that time, ask yourself: *What is asking for my attention, and what is asking to be released?* Listen without judgment, and then be open to making space for change.

What will you create space for in your life today?

MIND OVER BODY

Your body is the servant of your mind.

Your body listens to your mind more than you may realize. Every thought, every belief, every emotion—your body receives each one like a command. When your mind is weighed down by fear, stress, or self-doubt, your body responds in kind: tense muscles, shallow breath, exhaustion. But when your thoughts are rooted in hope, clarity, and self-respect, your body shifts, relaxing, energizing, aligning.

This connection between mind and body is foundational to our overall health and wellness. We can train for hours, eat well, and follow the "perfect" routine, but if our minds are working against us, our progress will stall. A discouraged mind can sabotage the strongest body, while an empowered mind can unlock resilience we didn't know we had. That's why inner fitness is just as vital as physical training. The most powerful transformations begin not with our bodies but with the thoughts we choose to believe.

Be mindful of your inner dialogue. Replace criticism with encouragement. Affirm your worth daily. Visualize strength. Speak life into your body. It is listening.

What thought do you need to shift in your mind today to better support your body?

THE ART OF COMMUNICATION

A whisper can reverberate like thunder,
while a shout can fade into silence.

The essence of communication goes far beyond the words we use. It lives in the pauses, in the tone of our voice, in the intention behind every syllable. A message delivered with care can comfort, empower, and inspire. But even the most well-meaning words, if rushed, forced, or thoughtless, can miss their mark.

We often think our voice's power lies in volume or eloquence. But in reality, the most impactful conversations are shaped by authenticity, presence, and emotional awareness. A quiet truth, gently spoken, can reach deeper than a loud declaration. A well-placed pause can offer more understanding than a thousand explanations.

Communication goes beyond making sure we're heard or that we got our point across. Real communication is about creating a space where clarity, respect, and connection can thrive. *Words are the brushstrokes, but the delivery is the final masterpiece.*

Be intentional with your words and the way in which you deliver them. Let your tone convey compassion, your silence carry presence, and your timing reflect wisdom. Communication is an everyday art—make each exchange one worth remembering.

How might the conversations in your life shift if you focused less on saying the right words and more on being real?

THE COURAGE TO HEAL

Healing means feeling the hurt and choosing to move forward with courage anyway.

Shame has a way of anchoring us to the past. It whispers that we're defined by what happened, by who we were, by the mistakes we made. Shame convinces us that moving forward is betrayal—that in healing we erase the pain, forget where we've come from. But real healing doesn't ask us to forget. Instead, we must face the wound with compassion—and then choose growth. You can acknowledge the past without living in it. You can carry the lessons without carrying the weight.

Healing begins the moment you stop letting shame make your decisions and start allowing courage to guide your steps. Every time you choose to rise up, to speak, to try again, to love despite the scar, you're rewriting your story. You're proving that wounds may shape you, but they don't have to define you.

Don't wait for pain to disappear before being willing to begin again. Start anyway. Move forward now. Your next chapter is already waiting.

What part of your past are you still letting shame hold hostage? What would it look like to release it with courage today?

SHOW UP READY

Those who lead don't just show up—they show up ready.

Effective leadership starts before you ever say a word or enter a room. Beyond just being present, it's about *how* you show up. Mentally sharp, emotionally steady, spiritually aligned.

The most impactful leaders aren't reactive—they're prepared. When we take time to ground ourselves—arriving early, clarifying our intention, aligning with our values—we bring a different energy into the space. Instead of scrambling to catch up, we're ready to lead with presence and purpose.

Leadership does not come from control or status. It's found in the daily practice of preparation, awareness, and consistency. And that practice begins long before the spotlight hits. It begins in the quiet moments—when no one is watching but everything is being shaped.

Being on time is the bare minimum. Start showing up early, and arrive focused, intentional, and fully ready. Whether you're preparing for a workout, a business meeting, or a meaningful conversation, take a few intentional minutes beforehand to align your purpose and energy.

What might some of your interactions look like if you chose to show up ready instead of just on time?

THE GIFT OF GOODBYE

When people walk away, it's often a hidden blessing, making space for something better.

It's easy to see someone's departure as a loss, as a crack in the foundation you trusted. But not everyone is meant to stay. Some people are chapters, not entire books. Some are stepping stones, not destinations.

When someone walks away, it can feel like rejection. But when that happens, it's simply the end of a chapter—not the end of your story. Not every relationship is meant to last forever. Some people enter our lives to teach us, to stretch us, to walk beside us for a while—and then their part is done. That doesn't mean the connection we had was meaningless. It simply means it served its season.

Letting go isn't failure. It's grace. It's trust. It's faith that what's ahead is greater than what's gone. The doors that close aren't the end of your story—they're the making of it.

Let go of what no longer serves you—without resentment. That empty space left behind isn't a loss; it's preparation. Trust that something more aligned, more honest, and more healing is already finding its way to you to fill you up.

Where in your life could you see a goodbye as a powerful new beginning?

THE WISDOM IN THE FOG

Uncertainty doesn't mean you're lost; it's often the space where something new is waiting to unfold.

When life feels unclear, your first instinct might be to push harder, to force your way through the fog to get to the other side. But uncertainty isn't always a problem you need to solve; it can be a signal to slow down. Fog doesn't always mean you're lost or on the wrong path. It may just mean you can't quite make out the path you're on. The next step, the next idea, the next version of you may need some quiet before what's forming can emerge into clarity.

Instead of rushing blindly ahead in the fog, choose to pause—listen to the quiet, feel the stillness, and begin to hear the whisper of clarity. Insight often arrives in subtle silence, not in the shout of speed. Growth isn't always loud or linear. Sometimes, the most powerful transformation happens in the space where you're simply willing to sit with what is.

If the road ahead seems unclear, resist the urge to sprint. Let yourself sit with the uncertainty. Trust that clarity is coming—but only if you give it the space to speak.

What wisdom might be waiting in the fog if you stopped rushing long enough to hear it?

STRENGTH IN SENSITIVITY

A sensitive mind isn't weak; it's highly aware. Use that awareness without letting it use you.

A sensitive mind is attuned to subtleties others may miss—a shift in tone, tension behind a smile, the unspoken energy in a room. Within that heightened awareness lives both a challenge and a gift. We can feel everything so deeply that it overwhelms, or we can channel our sensitivity into empathy, creativity, intuition, and insight.

Many view sensitivity as something to fix, as if it reflects a lack of strength. But a deeply sensitive mind is quick to perceive, intensely aware of its surroundings and the emotions of others. Sensitivity is not a flaw; it's actually a form of intelligence.

It's time to stop fighting our sensitivity and start working with it. Breathwork, movement, and mindfulness can transform anxious energy into clarity, focus, and wisdom. What once felt like a burden can become a source of empathy and insight. The key is not silencing your sensitivity but honoring it and embracing its strength.

Do you feel like your mind runs fast or feels too much? Pause and reframe: *How can this sensitivity serve me rather than cause me to suffer?* With the right tools, your anxious mind can become a quiet superpower.

What might change if you stopped seeing your sensitivity as a problem and started seeing it as a gift?

DRIVE MEETS DISCIPLINE

Without drive, discipline becomes a hollow routine, motion without meaning.

Sometimes everything looks right on the surface you're putting in consistent effort, you've set clear goals, you're making steady progress. From the outside, this looks like discipline. But inside? You might feel empty. Because discipline without drive is just going through the motions.

Discipline keeps you afloat; it keeps you moving—but it doesn't move you forward *with meaning*. Drive breathes soul into the structure of discipline. Drive is the purpose behind the plan, the reason behind the routine. When you're fueled by something deeper—a mission, a vision, a powerful *why*—discipline transforms. Instead of a grind, it becomes devotion.

The work may stay the same. The patterns and efforts might not change. But the energy behind them changes everything. That inner shift into *drive* transforms effort into impact.

Take a moment today to reconnect with the reason behind your routine. Why are you doing what you do? Are your daily efforts leading you somewhere that truly matters to you? If not, it's time to realign. Purpose fuels progress—and without it, even the most consistent effort can fall flat.

What's the deeper reason behind your discipline? Is it strong enough to keep you going?

JUNE 13

EMOTIONS ARE MESSENGERS

Emotions aren't our master. They are messengers asking to be acknowledged, not obeyed.

Emotions are part of what make us beautifully human. They give color to our experiences, help us understand our needs, and allow us to connect more deeply with others. But when emotions are driving the bus, they can cloud our judgment, distort our perception, and sabotage whatever progress we're trying to make.

Perhaps you've had moments when anger led you to say things you didn't mean, fear kept you from stepping into something you were ready for, or resentment held you back from reconciliation. These responses don't make you weak—they make you *human*, following the lead of your emotions.

But emotions aren't meant to control us. Emotions are meant to *guide* us. Like waves, they rise and fall. If we're paying attention, emotions offer signals that help us make meaningful decisions. Our strength lies in learning to listen to them with awareness and grace.

> The next time you feel overwhelmed, name what you're feeling. Put some space between the emotion and whatever action you might want to take. Allow yourself to feel whatever it is that's coming up, and then determine how you will move through it.

What are your emotions trying to tell you? How can you respond with clarity instead of reacting out of habit?

WHEN FEAR KNOCKS

It is better to understand fear than to numb it.

Many people spend their lives trying to outrun fear, burying it beneath distraction, ambition, or denial. But fear doesn't go away just because we ignore it. Instead of seeing fear as a threat, what if we looked at it as a guide? Many times, fear is signaling something deeper: a boundary we need to push, a truth we've been avoiding, a wound asking to be healed.

Our relationship with fear and our ability to listen can reframe how we respond to feelings of fear. When we embrace the courage to understand our fear rather than suppressing it, we unlock valuable insight. That awareness becomes the key that opens the door to new insight and understanding.

When we face what unsettles us, we can begin to reclaim power, clarity, and direction.

> When fear surfaces, don't rush to silence it. Pause and ask: *What is this fear trying to show me? What is beneath this fear?* You may find your fear is actually a mirror that reflects a deeper need. Understanding fear doesn't mean it goes away, but it does mean you're no longer controlled by it.

How will you respond the next time fear knocks on your door?

THE MOMENTS THAT MATTER

What fills the heart isn't screen time—it's the moments we dare to share together.

We live in a world of endless pings, posts, and priorities. Devices keep us informed and connected, yet they can also keep us distant—from others, from ourselves, from the present moment. The calendar may be full, but when we look back, the inbox and schedule won't be what we remember. We'll remember the spontaneous laughter, the look in another person's eyes, the quiet evening spent without distraction.

These are the moments that linger—the ones where presence replaced productivity, where connection took precedence over convenience. True fulfillment isn't found in the number of messages sent or tasks checked off. It's in the stories we co-create, the love we share, and the time we choose to give others—fully and freely.

Set down your phone. Look someone in the eye. Listen with your full attention. Create space for the unplanned and the meaningful. The world behind your screen can wait, but the people in front of you can't.

What's one meaningful moment you've missed—or nearly missed—because you were caught in the noise of the digital world? How can you show up more fully today?

THE STRENGTH OF STILLNESS

Mastering emotional boxing doesn't require counterpunches or fancy footwork; just standing still amid the storm is enough.

When emotions flare or criticism flies, your first instinct might be to react—to defend yourself, prove a point, or strike back. But true emotional strength is found in restraint rather than retaliation. Stillness isn't silence born of fear; it's presence rooted in power. It's choosing not to be pulled into someone else's chaos, not because you're weak but because you're wise.

You don't need to win every argument to win your peace. You don't need to counter every jab to protect your worth. Standing still amid emotional turbulence doesn't mean you're disconnected. It means you're in control.

It's easy to fight. It takes real courage to hold your ground, breathe, and let the moment pass without becoming part of the rumble. The gift of stillness requires strength.

The next time tensions rise, choose stillness. Don't get swept into the emotional ring. Stay rooted in your truth. The strongest response isn't always a louder voice, but rather a calm that refuses to become disturbed. Let stillness be your strength. Let peace be your power.

What would staying grounded—rather than reacting—allow you to protect within yourself?

EMBRACE THE DANCE

It's better to be worn out from dancing with life than rusty from standing still.

Life is movement. And yet how often do we hesitate, waiting for the perfect moment, the flawless plan, the guaranteed outcome? But waiting rarely delivers clarity. Instead, it often leads to stagnation, missed opportunities, and untapped potential. Because life doesn't reward perfection—it rewards participation.

Taking action, even imperfectly, breathes energy into our days. Each step forward—every risk, every stumble—adds rhythm to the dance of life. We don't grow by thinking about the next move but by taking it. When we're in motion, momentum builds. As momentum builds, clarity surfaces—clarity of purpose, of direction, of knowing what matters most. And as that clarity takes the lead, we discover the richness of a life fully lived.

You may fall sometimes. But keep dancing anyway, especially when the music of possibility is playing.

Don't let fear or overthinking keep you on the sidelines. Take that first step. Try that new thing. Embrace motion. Even if your steps aren't perfectly placed or timed, you're still living, growing, moving, and discovering what you're capable of. Life is meant to be experienced!

Where in your life have you been standing still? What one small step can you take today to start dancing again?

BELIEFS AND REALITY

Your beliefs may feel right, but do they match reality?

Our beliefs shape the way we move through the world. They influence our thoughts, decisions, and how we perceive others and ourselves. But not all beliefs are rooted in truth—some are born from fear, past wounds, or stories we've repeated so often that they feel like facts. Just because a belief feels familiar, that doesn't mean it's accurate. When we cling too tightly to untested beliefs, we risk building our lives on illusion.

Growth requires curiosity, the willingness to ask: *Is this belief serving me or limiting me?* The strongest people aren't those with unwavering certainty but those with the courage to question what they've always believed. Because the moment we begin to challenge our assumptions, we step closer to clarity, freedom, and transformation.

Pause today and examine a belief you've never questioned. Does it hold up in the light of truth? Does it align with who you want to become? Let go of what no longer serves your growth. The truth may be uncomfortable, but it is also liberating.

Which belief are you willing to reexamine in order to create a clearer, freer path forward?

THE IRONY OF WANTING

Desire is both the fuel that drives us and the fire that burns us—the difference lies in intention.

Desire is that inner spark that drives us to grow, create, and rise beyond where we stand now. Desire is where dreams live. Desire can lift you up or weigh you down. When your wants are anchored in purpose and clarity, they serve as a compass, pointing you toward meaningful progress. But when desire is fueled by comparison, fear, or scarcity, it can become a trap, pulling you into frustration, exhaustion, or even self-sabotage. You've likely felt both: the fire that moves you forward and the burn that leaves you spent. The difference lies in intention.

Wanting something isn't wrong. It's a natural part of our makeup. But when you learn to want *wisely*, you'll find your power. Learn to ask yourself: *Is this desire aligned with who I truly am, or am I chasing something that's leading me away from myself?*

Pause and reflect on what you're currently chasing. Is it fueling your purpose or burning you out? Is it lifting you up or weighing you down? Let your desire lead you, but don't allow it to own you.

What are you wanting right now? Is it leading you toward fulfillment or further away from yourself?

YOUR HOMECOMING

Growth isn't about becoming someone new but instead uncovering more of who you've always been.

Transformation doesn't mean abandoning who you are. It's about returning to who you've always been at the core. We are born as unique beings, filled with abilities, hopes, and dreams. And then life adds layers: Expectations, fears, comparisons, and survival strategies slowly bury your essence beneath the demands of the world.

You may think that growth means becoming someone else—an individual who is stronger, smarter, more accomplished. But the deepest growth often comes when we stop trying to add more and instead begin the process of unlearning, releasing, and remembering. As we begin peeling back layers instead of piling them on, we begin to honor the parts of ourselves that had once been silenced.

Real evolution isn't a reinvention. It's a return—a homecoming to your truest self.

Take a quiet moment to reflect: *What parts of myself have been buried under pressure, fear, or performance?* Rather than striving to become someone new, ask yourself who you were before the world told you who to be. Let growth be an unfolding, not a reconstruction. Honor your evolution by showing up more fully as yourself. Real freedom and growth are just beginning.

Who are you ready to rediscover beneath the surface?

JUNE 21

THE WEIGHT OF HOLDING ON

Holding on can hurt more than letting go.

There often comes a time when the weight of holding on is heavier than the fear of letting go. Whether it's a relationship, a dream, or a version of yourself that no longer fits, letting go isn't weakness—it's wisdom. Choosing to let go doesn't mean you didn't care. It means you care about your peace so much that you're willing to stop clinging to what no longer serves you.

True strength lies in loosening your grip. You're not giving up—you're making space for healing, growth, and something more aligned. Rather than erasing the past, you're honoring it by taking what you need, learning, and choosing to move forward. When you surrender, you find your freedom. What's meant for you will never require you to break. Peace begins where pressure ends.

> What are you gripping out of fear, and what's quietly holding you back? Not everything is meant to be carried. Breathe into the discomfort. Loosen your hold—not because it's easy but because you're ready to let go. Release what no longer aligns, and reclaim the space to be free.

What are you still holding on to that's already let go of you? What could open up in your life if you finally gave yourself permission to release it?

THE COST OF REVENGE

Revenge doesn't help you settle the score—
you instead inherit the other's burden.

We often fall prey to the powerful illusion that revenge will restore justice or heal wounds. But in truth, revenge only deepens pain. Carrying resentment is like clutching a burning coal—hoping to hurt another but scorching your own hand instead.

The pursuit of payback keeps us tethered to the very pain we wish to escape. The more you fixate on retribution, the more space you give to anger, bitterness, and the past. Letting go isn't about condoning wrongs or forgetting what happened. It's about freeing yourself. It's about choosing peace over poison and allowing healing to begin.

Releasing the grip of vengeance isn't a sign of weakness—it's the ultimate strength. Because moving forward on *your* path with clarity and self-respect requires far more courage than holding on to the pain.

If you've been holding on to resentment, pause and ask yourself: *Is this weight helping me grow or holding me back?* Choose forgiveness—not for the other person's benefit but for your own liberation. You don't need to carry someone else's burden. Let go, and reclaim the emotional space revenge once occupied.

What burden of the past are you ready to release so you can reclaim your peace today?

BUILD MORE THAN MUSCLE

Physical strength may fade, but wisdom and integrity will carry you for life.

Many of us are chasing physical excellence, believing that strength, appearance, and control over our bodies will unlock fulfillment. If we look the part, if we're at peak performance, we reason, life will somehow fall into place.

But time has a way of revealing what surface strength and appearance can't teach. Muscle doesn't prepare you for heartbreak. Abs don't teach you empathy. Biceps won't help you navigate loss or forgive when it feels impossible. What carries us through life's storms is deeper: our mind-set, our values, our compassion.

Physical strength will fade with time, but integrity, wisdom, and character strengthen with age—if we choose to nurture them. So yes, work for physical health and performance, but don't forget that what people will remember is the weight you helped them carry when life was hard.

As you're training your body, don't neglect what's inside. Feed your mind. Reflect on who you want to be. Act in alignment with your values just as fiercely as you train your muscles. Because one day, when the passage of time has worn down your outer self, your character, your purpose, and your integrity will continue to stand strong.

What are you doing today to build up the parts of yourself that truly last?

INTEGRITY IS THE LIGHT

Integrity reveals itself in the choices you make when no one is watching.

The right path often feels like the hardest one. Cutting corners feels harmless. Silence seems less risky than speaking truth. A small lie looks like it will protect something bigger. Taking undeserved credit would be a boost.

But doing the wrong thing, even if you can convince yourself it's for the right reason, is still wrong. Outcomes don't reveal integrity—your choices and actions do. Each time you choose truth over convenience, values over approval, honesty over ease, you strengthen the foundation of who you are. Even if no one else notices, *you* will know. And that quiet knowing—the knowledge that you stand firm when it matters—is a power that cannot be taken from you.

The light of integrity doesn't blind—it guides. And the people who matter most to you will feel its warmth, even if they never say a word.

The next time you face a decision that tests your truth, ask yourself: *Will this choice honor the person I'm becoming?* Choose integrity—not because it's easy but because it's who you are.

Where are you being asked to choose between easy and right? How would it feel to choose what aligns with your values?

THE ESSENCE OF JOY

Happiness is felt, not held.

There are times when we try to hold tightly to happiness, afraid it might slip away if we don't grasp it hard enough or that we'll never have access to it again. We think if we can just freeze this moment, we'll be able to make our joy last forever. But joy doesn't work that way. It isn't something we can control or capture or possess.

Happiness lives in presence—in laughter, stillness, connection, and breath. It flows most freely when we stop chasing it and simply allow ourselves to *feel* it. The more we try to grip it, the more distant it becomes. But when we relax into the moment, without fear or attachment, happiness shows up like sunlight breaking through clouds—warm, radiant, and enough.

Joy doesn't need to be held. It needs only to be welcomed.

Give yourself permission to feel joy today without needing to own it or trying to make it last forever. Don't chase joy or cling to it. Instead, show up fully for the small moments that bring you peace, laughter, and beauty. Trust that joy will return again and again, in different forms.

Where can you soften your grip today and allow happiness to simply flow?

THE LEGACY OF TRUE LEADERSHIP

True leaders don't just inspire others. They teach the people they're leading how to inspire themselves.

The best leaders don't create dependency—they create self-leaders.

We often look to leaders for direction, hoping to be pushed or pulled into action. But the leaders who make the most lasting impact don't feed us answers. Instead, they help us find our own. They show us how to trust our instincts, make decisions with confidence, and believe in our own strength. Their leadership isn't loud and commanding; it's quiet and empowering.

True leadership is not about standing in front of the person you're leading but walking beside them. It's about helping others ignite the fire within so they can keep going long after you're gone.

If you find yourself in a position to lead—at home, at work, or in your community—ask yourself: *Am I trying to be the light, or am I helping others find their own light?* Commit to empowering those around you. Share your tools, your wisdom, and most importantly, your belief in their potential. Leadership is about more than what you achieve. It's about the legacy you leave in the people who rise up because of your influence.

Who in your life can you empower to lead themselves today?

THE FREEDOM OF LOVE

Love rooted in ego is actually attachment dressed in disguise. True love flows from freedom, not control.

Ego says, "You complete me." Love says, "You are already whole." When we confuse attachment for love, we cling—not because we care deeply but because we fear deeply. Attachment is love distorted by insecurity. It seeks to possess, to control, to define another through our own unmet needs.

But real love doesn't demand. It respects. Love doesn't shrink the other person but instead celebrates their growth. True love arises not from the fear of losing someone but from the freedom to let them be fully themselves—even if that means they grow in directions we didn't expect.

Love isn't about holding tighter. It's about holding space. The difference between love and attachment is the difference between empowerment and entanglement.

Look closely at how you love. Ask yourself: *Am I offering freedom, or am I seeking control?* Loosen your grip. Allow love to breathe, to evolve, to flow without fear. Love that is free is the only kind that truly lasts.

What would shift in your relationships if you loved without needing to hold on so tightly?

THE WEIGHT OF THE PAST

If you chain the present to the past, you silence the whispers of new beginnings.

You can't rewrite the past, but you can stop allowing the past to write your present. The longer you carry the weight of old mistakes, regrets, or missed chances, the more you miss out on the quiet invitations of what's possible now.

The past has its purpose, but it was never meant to take up permanent residence in your mind. When you dwell too long on what was, you risk missing what is and what could be. Maybe it shows up as refusing to try again because last time you failed. Or holding back trust because someone once betrayed you. Or staying silent because your voice wasn't valued before.

Your next chapter can't unfold if you're still rereading the last one. Growth begins the moment you choose to loosen your grip on the weight of the past and make space for something new.

What are you still holding that no longer serves you? Guilt? Shame? A story that keeps you small? Breathe into the present. Release what weighs you down. There is power in choosing to begin again.

What would become possible if you stopped letting your past define your now?

WHEN THE MAP BURNS

When your map burns, don't give up.
Look for a new way forward.

We all begin with a plan—a path we think will carry us to the life we envision for ourselves. But what happens when that plan crumbles? What happens when the map burns and the familiar path we so carefully plotted disappears into uncertainty? Those painful moments are invitations—not to quit but to evolve.

A burned map doesn't mean the journey is over—it means it's time to lead with intuition rather than instruction. Your goal hasn't vanished. Your mission hasn't changed. The route you'll take to get there is simply different now. And sometimes that detour becomes a defining—and refining—chapter along the journey.

Growth happens when we rise up and move forward, even when our plan falls apart.

> If you're staring at a pile of ashes, don't mourn the map—ignite a new path forward. Let your values guide your steps. Let your heart remind you of what still matters. You don't need a perfect plan to keep going; you just need the will to move forward.

What dream or vision calls to you, even if your map has burned? What will you do to take the next step?

COME HOME TO *NOW*

If you're lost in that middle place called *elsewhere*, remember that nothing is more real than the present.

It's easy to get caught between two illusions—the past you can't change and the future that hasn't yet arrived. Perhaps you keep replaying old mistakes or worrying about what's ahead, thinking that either might give you control or answers.

But your true power lives here, in the *now*. This moment—today, the present—is where you make decisions, find peace, and begin to grow. When you stop dwelling on the past and worrying about the future, your awareness of the present—even if only for a breath—allows you to slow down, see clearly, and reconnect with what matters.

The present isn't a stepping stone to something better. *The present is the destination.* Life isn't waiting for you to arrive. It's unfolding right now in front of your eyes. Will you choose to show up for it?

> Pause and take a deep breath. Look around. Ask yourself: *Am I here, in the present, or am I lost elsewhere?* Return to this moment with intention. No matter what has occurred or what lies ahead, you can always come home to *now*. This very moment is where life begins, peace takes root, and transformation becomes possible.

How will you return to the present in your life today?

JULY

LETTING GO OF ANGER

You have the power to choose to carry or release your anger.

Anger is often seen as a response to someone else's actions. But in truth, anger lives inside us. It may be sparked by injustice, betrayal, or pain, but the flame is ours to fuel or extinguish. Holding on to anger might feel like protection, a way to reclaim control or assert power. But over time, anger hardens into resentment and the weight becomes ours to bear.

Letting go of anger isn't about dismissing our pain or excusing the offense. Instead, it's about choosing not to let pain continue to damage your peace. It's a conscious decision to stop carrying the burden and allow space for healing.

You can embrace the liberation of peace regardless of circumstances—because the one who releases anger frees themself first.

Take a quiet moment to reflect. Have you been holding on to anger—toward another, toward a situation, or even toward yourself? Breathe into that space. Acknowledge it without shame. Then ask: *What would it feel like to let this go?* The door to peace is already open. You need only the courage to walk through it.

What's one small way you can begin releasing the anger that no longer serves your peace?

"NO" IS A COMPLETE SENTENCE

No means no. No explanation, justification, or exceptions required.

One of the most powerful acts of self-respect we can practice is setting a boundary—and honoring it. This isn't always easy. In the interest of wanting to please others, avoid conflict, or be understood and appreciated, we over-explain, soften our "no," or allow guilt to override what we know to be right for us.

But the cost of not setting and keeping boundaries is real. Our peace, our energy, and sometimes even our sense of self are on the line. The moment we realize that "no" is a complete sentence and embrace it, everything begins to shift. We stop diluting our needs and start standing by them with conviction and care. And the more we practice that, the more we give others permission to do the same.

Boundaries don't close us off from others. Boundaries are threads, stitching up healthier relationships grounded in mutual respect.

Practice saying no with clarity and without guilt. Whether you're declining an invitation, protecting your rest, or stepping away from something that doesn't align with your values, let your boundary stand. Saying no isn't rude or selfish. It's a declaration of self-respect. And when you honor your boundaries, you give others permission to honor theirs.

How can you honor your boundaries today without apology?

RISE UP FOR JUSTICE

The scales of equality won't tip themselves.
We must fight for equality for all.

Equality isn't a gift, bestowed by some unseen force or benefactor. Equality is something we need to be fighting for daily. For too long, society has drawn lines where there should have been bridges. Gender, race, identity, ability, and economic status have all been used as silent gatekeepers to opportunity. And though awareness has grown, injustice hasn't vanished.

The scales are still tilted, and balance doesn't happen by chance. True equality means taking action, leveling the field so that *everyone*—regardless of background or identity—has an equal chance to rise, to speak, to lead, to live with dignity.

This work toward equality and justice isn't just for the marginalized. It belongs to all of us. Because silence is a stance. And neutrality, in the face of inequality, protects the imbalance.

Ask yourself a hard question: *Am I contributing to justice or simply coexisting with injustice?* Speak up when it's uncomfortable. Listen when a conversation or issue isn't about you. Use your position—whatever that may be—to amplify fairness. The scales won't tip themselves. And equality won't rise unless we rise with it—loud, united, and unshakably committed.

How will you stand up today for those fighting to be seen and heard?

FROM FEAR TO FREEDOM

Understanding your fear will help you step into bigger and better things in the future.

Fear is often misunderstood. One common misconception is that fear is weakness, but it's not—it's a signal. A teacher. A mirror reflecting where we feel uncertain, unready, or unworthy. You may have shrunk in fear's shadow yesterday. But growth starts the moment you stop running from fear and start *listening* to it.

Understanding fear transforms it. When you ask, *Why am I afraid?* you shift from wandering to being a guide. You begin to see patterns. You connect past wounds to present hesitations. And what once paralyzed you can suddenly become a path forward.

Fear won't vanish overnight. But clarity and understanding about why it has such a hold on you will weaken its grip. Each layer of awareness will build trust in your next step—and that trust will turn into freedom. The future isn't something to fear. It's something to *claim.*

Instead of trying to silence or ignore fear, interrogate it. Sit with it. Learn from it. Then move forward, not without fear but with the wisdom it has given you.

What fear have you outgrown? How will that freedom help you take bolder steps tomorrow?

FREEDOM FOR ALL

Freedom is more than autonomy. True freedom is the presence of choice, voice, and dignity.

Freedom isn't simply about removing barriers. It's about creating space for authenticity. Freedom is what allows us to choose our path, speak our truth, and live with self-respect. True freedom empowers—not just the individual but the collective. Living a life of freedom isn't one of reckless abandon; it's conscious liberation. Freedom asks us to own our choices, to use our voice courageously, and to walk in alignment with our values.

But freedom isn't just individual. Freedom is collective. It's relational. When we use our freedom to uplift others, we become stewards of dignity and protectors of justice. Freedom that isolates becomes entitlement. Freedom that includes becomes legacy.

Every time you choose truth over silence, empathy over judgment, or courage over conformity, you model what freedom can be. And in doing so, you light the path for others.

Don't just enjoy your freedom. Embody it! Advocate for freedom in the places where it is denied. Extend it when you see that it has been withheld. Choose not only what serves you but also what honors humanity as a whole.

How can you use your freedom today to create more dignity, voice, and space for yourself and for others?

EMBRACE YOUR BECOMING

You are capable and worthy and are already becoming the person you're meant to be.

It's easy to believe that who we're meant to become lies somewhere in the distance, that we have to earn it or prove ourselves somehow. But *becoming* isn't about reaching some final, polished version of ourselves. It's the journey of transformation that happens in the present, at this very moment.

Every choice, every setback, every small act of courage contributes to who we are becoming right now. The process isn't reserved until everything looks perfect, until all the stars are aligned. Where we are right this minute—with all our doubts, efforts, fears, failings, and hopes—is the daily unfolding of growth in each of us. We are all becoming, right now.

Take a moment to reflect on how far you've come—not just in what you've achieved, but in how you've grown through every experience. Let go of the belief that you need to become someone else to be worthy. *You* are already in motion. Show up for yourself today with grace and belief. There is no "next version" of you. There is only you—the ever-evolving, continuously growing, and constantly becoming *you*, which is enough—right here and right now.

How will you honor your journey of becoming today?

THE STRENGTH BENEATH THE SCAR

Though the emotional scars of past wounds may remain, they often become quiet sources of strength.

Scars aren't signs of brokenness. Scars reveal that we've healed. They're evidence that something tried to stop us—and failed. While emotional wounds may not leave visible marks, they shape us just the same. Those healed scars are etched into the heart, quietly guiding how we love, trust, and move through the world. At first, these scars may be tender. But over time, they soften, becoming gentle reminders of our strength and survival.

What once felt like pain becomes a source of perspective.

What once brought us to our knees now stands as a testament to our endurance.

Our scars become teachers—offering lessons in compassion, empathy, and the quiet kind of courage that comes from facing the storm and choosing to rise anyway.

> Don't hide your scars. Honor them. Let them reveal not just what hurt you but, more importantly, what *healed* you. Allow your scars to remind you of the fire you walked through and the strength that got you through the flames. You aren't defined by the pain but by the resilience you summoned in its aftermath.

Which of your scars can you now see as a badge of strength?

THE BEST WORKOUT INTENSITY

What's the best workout intensity? The one you'll stick with—tomorrow, and the day after that.

In the fitness world, intensity often grabs all the attention. You're told to push harder, go longer, sweat more—until you're sore, drained, or even injured. It's easy to believe that only extreme effort will lead to real results.

Lasting transformation doesn't come from the workouts that break you but from the ones you can *sustain*. The sessions that truly shape body and mind aren't always the hardest—they're the ones you return to. They become part of your rhythm, part of your life.

Physical health and fitness aren't about punishing yourself. True fitness comes from honoring your body with consistent, intentional effort—through mindful daily choices that support your body's needs and create a sustainable lifestyle you can embrace for years to come.

It's time to rethink what intensity really means. You don't have to push yourself to the edge every time to get stronger. Aim for workouts that challenge instead of deplete you. Choose movement that leaves you feeling empowered, not exhausted. Create a rhythm that fits your life, fuels your energy, and moves you steadily toward your goals.

What pace can you commit to—not just today but for the long run?

THE COMPASS WITHIN

When your mind creates labyrinths of uncertainty, remember that your heart holds a compass that needs no map.

The mind can be a maze—full of loops, second-guessing, and the constant pressure to find the "right" answer. It wants clarity, guarantees, logic. But when you're standing at a crossroads and nothing makes sense, your mind doesn't lead you forward. Your heart does.

Your heart doesn't deal in details. It doesn't explain or justify. It just *knows*. It speaks in quiet pulls and subtle truths. And while the mind may demand a map, the heart offers direction—not by telling you, "Walk ten paces north," but by providing meaning.

This is the deeper wisdom—the kind that's felt, not forced. Trusted, not logically proven. When the noise of uncertainty grows too loud, your job isn't to solve everything or have all the answers. It's to quiet the outside chaos just enough to hear the whisper within that gently says, *This way.*

When doubt crowds your path, pause. Close your eyes. Breathe into your body. Let your heart speak—and dare to follow where it leads.

Where have you been overthinking your next move?
What truth is your heart trying to tell you?

THE BALANCE OF LOVE

Jealousy in love is like trying to hold on to water.
The tighter the grip, the faster it escapes.

Love isn't meant to be possessed—it's meant to be shared, nurtured, and respected. Yet many fall into the trap of control, mistaking it for protection. Jealousy often stems from fear: fear of loss, fear of not being enough, fear of vulnerability. But trying to hold on to someone too tightly can suffocate the very thing you hope to preserve.

Real love breathes freely. It thrives in trust and grows stronger when space is honored and individuality is respected. True connection isn't built on ownership but on presence. It means offering space for another to grow while standing confidently in your own worth. Whether in romantic relationships, friendships, or family dynamics, when love is given—not demanded—it transforms from something fragile into something expansive.

If you notice yourself clinging out of fear, pause and ask yourself: *Am I protecting love, or am I trying to control it?* Release your grip and redirect your energy toward building trust, understanding, and mutual growth. Love isn't something to cage; it's something to cultivate.

Where in your relationships can you release control and invite in more freedom, trust, and connection?

LIFE OUTSIDE THE SCREEN

The world is 3D, not HD. Go out and enjoy it.

We live in a hyperconnected age, and it's easy to get swept up in the scroll—comparing our behind-the-scenes to everyone else's highlight reel. We mistake carefully curated moments for reality, forgetting that real life happens beyond the frame.

The most meaningful moments aren't captured—they're *lived.* They happen in laughter that isn't rehearsed, in deep conversations, in ordinary moments that feel extraordinary simply because we're fully present for them. Life in real time is messy, unpredictable, and breathtakingly honest. And that's where true joy lives—not in the likes but in the living. Screens may reflect pieces of life, but they'll never replace the richness of actually experiencing it.

Challenge yourself today to unplug and reconnect, with nature, people, and yourself. Step outside. Look someone in the eyes. Touch the earth. Laugh without recording it. Listen without distraction. You'll find that reality, with all its imperfections, is more vivid and rewarding than anything high definition can offer. If you want to feel fully alive, step into the real world—it's waiting for you.

When was the last time you truly experienced life, purely and wholly, without a screen filtering it?

THE LANDSCAPE WITHIN

Nothing is as secret as the depths of your own mind.

The richest and most mysterious journey we'll ever take is the one that leads inward. Beneath the noise of daily life, your mind holds layers of untapped insight, unresolved emotions, and silent truths. It's where fears hide, dreams whisper, and identity quietly takes shape.

Many people spend a lifetime navigating the outer world yet avoid exploring the vast terrain within. But real transformation begins when you dare to go inward—not to judge, but to understand. The parts of us we suppress—old wounds, limiting beliefs, inner doubts—don't vanish. They wait to be acknowledged. And when we meet them with honesty and compassion, something powerful happens—clarity deepens, strength resurfaces, and we become more fully ourselves.

This exercise isn't about fixing the mind but about *listening* to it, because your mind holds the blueprint of your becoming.

Take a moment to reflect today—not to solve but to see. Notice your patterns. Trace your beliefs. Give your inner world the same attention you give the outer one. There's a good chance that the answers you're seeking exist within.

What part of your inner world have you been avoiding? What might shift if you explored it with curiosity instead of fear?

JULY 13

THE FIRST RIPPLE

Change starts within. Heal yourself first, then your family, your community, and finally the world.

It's tempting to look outward when we want to make an impact—to fix what's broken, to heal what's hurting. But true change doesn't begin out there. It begins inside. It starts the moment you choose to heal your own wounds, challenge your own patterns, and nurture your own growth.

When you heal yourself, it naturally affects how you show up for others. You listen differently. You love differently. You lead differently. Your energy shifts, and that shift becomes a ripple—a quiet, powerful force that moves outward gently, without agenda.

You don't have to save the world all at once. You just have to start where you are. The healing process begins with just one ripple. From that center, the impact will expand into something strong, true, and lasting.

Turn inward today. Ask yourself: *Where do I need healing?* Begin there. Trust that even the smallest act of self-repair carries the power to reach far beyond you.

What is one area within you that, if healed, could create a ripple of change in your family, your community, or the world?

BECOMING ON THE WAY

The road to success can feel long and lonely, but every step holds a valuable lesson.

The path to success often looks nothing like we imagined. It winds; it climbs; it tests. There are stretches when progress feels invisible, when effort feels pointless, and when the silence makes us question everything.

But beneath the surface, something powerful is happening. We are *becoming*. We aren't simply achieving; we are evolving, growing, getting stronger and wiser. Each obstacle teaches resilience. Each pause invites reflection. And each step forward—no matter how small—builds the character needed to be trusted with whatever it is you're working toward.

Success isn't just the finish line. It's the transformation that happens along the way. You don't wake up one day ready—you grow ready. And often it's the unseen work, done in solitude, that prepares you most for the moment you've been chasing.

Stay committed to the process—even when it's quiet, even when the reward feels distant. You are being shaped by each challenge and each choice.

Who are you becoming through this journey? What parts of you are quietly growing stronger each day?

JULY 15

THE COURAGE TO BELIEVE

Embrace the courage to face the storm while still believing the sun will rise after it's over.

Positivity is often mistaken for denial—as if to be hopeful, we must turn a blind eye to pain or struggle. But real positivity is forged in fire. It's not the absence of difficulty but the presence of unwavering belief. It's choosing to stand in the storm, soaked and trembling, and still hold space for the promise of light. Positivity is not about forcing a smile when your heart is aching—it's about trusting that your strength is bigger than your circumstances.

The most powerful kind of optimism isn't loud. It's quiet and patient. It doesn't ignore the darkness—it walks through it with courage, knowing that hard times won't last forever. It says, "I don't know how or when, but I believe that better days are ahead." That belief is the anchor in life's rough waters.

When challenges weigh heavily on your shoulders, pause. Feel what's real. Then reach inward and find the courage to believe, not in perfection but in possibility.

What hope are you willing to hold on to today, even in the midst of the storm?

LISTEN TO THE FIRE

Purpose is the fire that keeps
burning when motivation fades.

Every meaningful journey will test you. Progress slows; setbacks shake your confidence; the path ahead may be unclear. In those moments, passion often flickers. But purpose? Purpose is a fire that stays lit. Purpose is the deeper *why* that lives beneath the goals, beyond the titles, away from the applause. Purpose is the foundation.

When you reconnect with the original spark of why you first started—what initially moved you, inspired you, woke you up—you will find fuel. Maybe it was the moment you knew you wanted to break a generational cycle. Or the first time you felt truly alive doing what you love. This fuel won't burn out quickly and fade. It will be solid and reliable, burning slow and steady through difficulty, distraction, and doubt.

Your inner fire is not lit by hype. It is stoked by clarity, consistency, and vision. When you nurture your *why*, you unlock a purpose that carries you, even when everything else says stop.

Reflect on what sparked your journey. What made you pursue this dream? Write it down. Speak it aloud. Let that fire remind you who you are and why you refuse to quit.

When the winds whip up and the road gets treacherous, what keeps you going?

BUILD YOUR OWN DESTINY

Your destination is your destiny, shaped by the choices you make.

While life can certainly surprise us, destiny itself is not random—it's shaped by our intention, integrity, and consistent action. Many believe that success comes from one breakthrough moment or lucky opportunity. Lightning-bolt moments do happen, but destiny is mostly something we build—in quiet, repeated, daily choices and actions. Each time we choose to keep going when it would be easier to quit, to speak up instead of staying silent, to take a step forward even when the path feels uncertain, we're building both a future *and* a foundation.

You can create your destiny by choosing to act in alignment with who you want to become. When you treat each moment as a step toward your desired future rather than waiting for some distant event to define you, you stop chasing destiny and start living it.

Look at where your life is headed, not through the lens of where you want to be but based on the choices you're making today. What small but meaningful step can you take today to move closer to the future you desire? Don't rely on chance. Build your destiny with intention, one choice at a time.

What decision could you make today that your future self will thank you for?

COURAGEOUS HONESTY

True honesty means being brave enough to be authentic, regardless of how you might be perceived.

Honesty is one of the most powerful and courageous acts we can practice. It's not about saying everything that's on your mind or being blunt just for the sake of it. True honesty is about being authentic when it matters most—showing up as your full self, even when it feels uncomfortable or scary. It means speaking the truth, not because it's easy but because it's right, and always delivering it with care and kindness.

But honesty isn't just about facts. It's about being transparent with your feelings, intentions, and boundaries. It means dropping the mask and trusting that truth matters more than being seen as perfect, agreeable, or easy.

Courageous honesty builds trust and strengthens connection—both with others and within us. It sparks richer conversations, clearer decisions, and more meaningful relationships. And it begins with self-honesty, acknowledging how you feel, what you need, and who you're becoming. When you choose to be real, you create space for others to do the same.

Speak your truth with intention and clarity. Listen with openness. Let honesty be the language upon which you build a life of authenticity and courage.

Where in your life is truth waiting to be spoken? What might shift if you finally voiced it?

JULY 19

THE DISGUISE OF CONTROL

When love turns to manipulation, it is no longer love.

Love is meant to be a safe haven built on trust, nurtured by mutual respect, and held together by freedom. But sometimes, what begins as love becomes entangled with fear, insecurity, or the desire to control. And that's when it begins to change. Subtle guilt, emotional pressure, or even silence used as punishment—these aren't expressions of love. They are signals that control has disguised itself as care.

Real love doesn't need tactics. It doesn't twist truth to "win" an argument or use affection as leverage. It communicates openly, supports freely, and honors the other's choices—especially when those choices are difficult. Manipulation, no matter how softly spoken or cleverly hidden, always leaves a trace of imbalance. And where manipulation lives, love cannot fully breathe.

Recognizing this shift takes courage, but it's the first step toward releasing control and reclaiming what real connection looks like.

Reflect on your relationships, both past and present. Have you experienced—or used—control disguised as love? Begin by choosing awareness and accountability. Let go of the need to shape others and, instead, love them in a way that gives them space to be themselves.

What does love without control look like in your life? Are you ready to choose it?

THE GIFT OF A PAUSE

Every stoplight is an opportunity to pause, breathe, and return to the present before life urges you forward again.

In a world that constantly urges us to go faster, do more, get more, we often overlook the value of slowing down. What we typically view as interruptions—red lights, long lines, brief moments of waiting—can actually be quiet invitations to pause. To breathe. To come back to ourselves.

These everyday pauses aren't wasted time. They're opportunities. When we resist our instinct to fill the blank space with words, with scrolling, with some kind of external input, we open the door for a moment of centering in the middle of our busy day. In those still moments, we can release tension, notice our thoughts, reconnect with the present, and remember that rushing isn't the same as living.

Life isn't just about forward motion—it's about awareness in motion. Sometimes the most meaningful progress begins with a single moment of stillness.

Honor the pauses that come across your path today. The next time life makes you wait, resist the urge to fill the silence, and instead *feel* the silence. Take one full breath. Let it bring you back to the moment. These pauses are hidden gifts, moments of needed stillness amid the chaos.

How will you use life's pauses to reconnect with the present starting right now?

REFLECTING THE LIGHT

Some search for flaws in others. Why not reflect their light instead?

It's easy to slip into the habit of looking for what's wrong—in ourselves, in others, in the world. Criticism is familiar; judgment becomes a default. But what if we flipped the script? What if, instead of searching for flaws, we became mirrors for the light that others already carry?

Every person carries something bright within them—kindness, resilience, creativity, humor. When we choose to reflect those traits back to them, we remind them of who they truly are. And in doing so, we often rediscover our own light. Reflecting the light doesn't mean ignoring imperfections. Instead, it means making a conscious decision to lead with encouragement rather than with critique. To see with eyes of compassion rather than comparison.

The more we reflect light, the more we multiply it. And in a world that often feels dimmed by division, that kind of intentional seeing becomes a quiet form of healing.

Pay attention to the light in others today. Acknowledge their gifts, speak to their strengths, and become a mirror for what is good and beautiful.

What kind of light will you reflect today? How might it shape someone's day?

MORE THAN HALF THE BATTLE

Showing up isn't half the battle—it's the key to breaking free from stagnation.

You may have heard the saying that showing up is half the battle—but that's only partly true. Showing up is *everything*. It's the key to overcoming the real struggle: the battle against stagnation, self-doubt, and delay. It's the foundation on which every breakthrough, every change, and every transformation is built. Without showing up—fully, consistently, and intentionally—true change doesn't stand a chance.

You don't need to have all the answers. You don't need the perfect plan. What you need is presence, commitment, and a willingness to face the moment as it is, even if you feel uncertain. Showing up says, "I'm here. I care. I'm in."

The most meaningful growth doesn't happen in grand gestures—it happens when you choose to show up on the hard days, the quiet days, the days when no one else is watching. That choice is where momentum lives. And that momentum is where change begins.

Decide today to show up for yourself with intention, with courage, and with consistency. It's the smallest step, but it holds enormous power.

Where in your life have you been waiting for the perfect moment to begin when all you really need to do is show up?

THE TRUTH BENEATH THE NOISE

Keep asking "Why?" until the answers run out. That's where the truth lives.

Truth isn't always the first answer. It's often the answer waiting beneath all the noise. Life is filled with distraction, opinion, and performance, and we can be quick to explain, justify, or defend. But when we pause and ask the simple question "Why?"—not just once, but again and again—we begin to peel back layers.

At first, we may meet surface-level answers, ones that have been shaped by habit or fear. But persistence brings us closer to what's real. Each *why* clears away another layer of noise until what remains is quiet, simple, and unshakably true. This truth isn't complicated. It won't shout. The voice of clarity has always been there, waiting beneath the clutter of expectation and assumption. And when we find it, more than answering the question, the truth anchors us.

If you're feeling unclear or off-center, pause and ask yourself why. Really ask yourself. Keep digging. Don't rush the process. The truth isn't found amid noise—it's revealed in the stillness just beyond it. Let your own questions guide you home.

What might you discover if you stayed curious long enough to find your deepest truth?

THE SEEDS OF TRIUMPH

The seeds of tomorrow's triumphs are often planted in the soil of today's struggles.

Injuries, failures, and disappointments often feel like setbacks—roadblocks standing in the way of the forward momentum we were expecting. But with time and perspective, it becomes clear that hardships aren't the end of the path; they're actually seeds that will grow into something strong and hardy.

Think of each challenge as a seed planted deep beneath the surface, preparing us for growth we can't yet see. Adversity stretches us—it tests our resilience, deepens our patience, and strengthens our self-belief. While it may not be obvious in the moment, the seeds are being watered and fertilized so that our greatest transformation can begin.

The strength we carry today was forged in yesterday's struggle. What may have felt like defeat was really preparation—soil being turned over for a future we're now ready to harvest.

Whatever you're facing today, trust that it has purpose. Struggle isn't a sign of weakness; it's a part of the growth process. Don't give up when things get hard. Instead, ask yourself: *What am I planting through this challenge?* Water it with perseverance, feed it with faith, and give it time to bloom into something stronger, deeper, and more meaningful.

What seeds are you planting today that future triumph will thank you for?

THE HIGH ACHIEVER'S MIND-SET

High achievers don't make excuses. They make plans, take action, and adjust until the goal becomes reality.

There is a common trait among those who consistently succeed: They don't let obstacles become excuses. High achievers may stumble, but they don't stay down for long. They don't wait for perfect timing or ideal conditions. Instead, they act—with clarity, purpose, and resilience.

Achievement isn't about having all the answers from the start. It's about taking initiative, learning along the way, and refusing to give up when things get tough. It's not about luck. It's not even about talent. It's about possessing a certain mind-set—one that sees setbacks as detours, not dead ends. The difference between dreaming and achieving often comes down to the willingness to show up, make a plan, and course-correct as needed.

> Take a hard look today at where you might be holding back. Are you offering excuses or building momentum? Choose one goal that matters to you. Write down a clear, simple plan. Take one action, no matter how small. And if that plan doesn't work? Adjust it. Stay committed. Your goal isn't a wish; it's a decision.

What's one excuse you can let go of today to get a step closer to your goal?

THE POWER OF SAYING "NOT NOW"

Every *no* is a *yes* to a priority you've already established.

So many of us have a hard time saying no. We don't want to disappoint or let someone down. We want to help, to deliver, to be seen as capable. But there's nothing wrong with saying, "Not now."

Not now is you making a *choice*. And choice is a form of power. In a world that glorifies hustle, it's easy to feel like every opportunity must be seized, every request answered, every task completed. But trying to do it all only leads to burnout and resentment. True strength lies in discernment, in recognizing what aligns with your energy, your values, and your season of life.

Saying "I don't have time right now" isn't a sign that you're falling short. Rather, making a mindful choice about your time is evidence that you're protecting what you've already deemed sacred. You're honoring your priorities, whether that's rest, presence, health, or focus. Saying no isn't selfish—it's strategic. Your *not now* is a boundary that safeguards what matters most.

Don't let guilt blur your clarity when deciding whether to commit to something. Say no when it serves your deeper yes. Let *not now* be a conscious act of alignment.

What are you truly saying yes to when you allow yourself to say no?

THE PATH TO WISDOM

Wisdom isn't found only in books and education. It is earned through experience.

Wisdom isn't only composed of everything that has been gathered in books, lectures, and the words of brilliant thinkers. That knowledge inspires and informs, but the kind of wisdom that shapes who we are at our core comes from lived experience, forged in the moments that test our patience, challenge our beliefs, and ask us to grow beyond who we were yesterday. The disappointments, the detours, the things that don't go as planned can be life's most profound classrooms.

Wisdom emerges not from theory, but from reflection. It's found in the meaning we choose to make of our hardest lessons. When we move through life with openness, courage, and a willingness to learn, we begin to realize that life itself is our greatest teacher. And the more present we are in each moment, the more wisdom we carry forward.

Instead of chasing more information, ask yourself: *What has life already taught me?* Embrace your journey—every setback, every success, every moment of growth. Allow your experiences to shape you, and turn reflection into your most powerful tool. Remember, wisdom doesn't come from knowledge; it comes from living with awareness.

What life lesson are you ready to turn into wisdom?

WHAT IS AUTONOMY?

True autonomy is the freedom to choose your path with responsibility, respect, and relationship.

Autonomy is often misunderstood. It isn't about going it alone, making all your decisions independently and without any input. Autonomy is a complex blend of the quiet strength of self-direction, living your values while respecting other people's journeys, not distancing yourself from others, and staying open to guidance while honoring your right to choose, act, and grow with intention.

When we respect autonomy—both ours and others'—we become more engaged, more confident, and more accountable for the lives we're building. In environments where autonomy is denied, creativity withers, trust erodes, and resentment grows. But when we embrace autonomy, freedom and responsibility rise hand in hand, inviting clarity, fostering integrity, and deepening connection.

Autonomy isn't a rebellion—it's a return to self. And when it's supported, people don't run away from others—they show up more fully for themselves and those around them.

Whether you're leading a team, raising a child, or reclaiming your own voice, choose to honor autonomy. Give space. Build trust. Invite collaboration, not control. When we stop managing every move and start empowering choice, we can help transform lives.

In what areas can you strengthen your autonomy? How might that shift your sense of purpose?

THE POWER OF AWARENESS

Awareness is the pause before taking a step, the moment of honesty that can change everything.

Awareness is often that thin line separating reaction from intention. So many of our choices—especially the ones we question later—are made on autopilot. We act from habit, from emotion, or from old stories without ever pausing to ask why.

But in that brief space between impulse and action lies incredible power. When we slow down before reaching for comfort, distraction, or escape, we begin to see what's really driving us: unmet needs, buried emotions, or misaligned priorities. That pause has the power to be a turning point. We won't get it right every time. But simply being present is a powerful first step.

With awareness, we have the power to stop repeating behaviors and start responding. We are able to act from clarity instead of conditioning. And even the smallest shift in consciousness can create a ripple of meaningful change.

The next time you feel compelled to act on an impulse, pause and ask yourself: *Why am I* really *doing this?* Don't judge. Just notice. That moment of truth can be the beginning of transformation.

What might change in your life if you started practicing deeper awareness?

SPEND YOUR ENERGY WISELY

Your greatest asset is your energy.
Focus it where it counts.

We can have hours at our disposal, but if our energy is scattered, nothing meaningful will take root. We all know the experience. We finally have a window of time to get something done, but instead of buckling down, our mind wanders, flitting from one low-value task to another. Before we know it, hours have passed and we haven't accomplished anything.

The key to success isn't how much time you have but how you show up during that time. When you protect your energy—setting boundaries, choosing where you invest your attention, saying no when needed—you gain clarity, direction, and momentum. You stop reacting and start creating. You act with intention rather than urgency. An hour fueled by focused energy will always outperform a full day of depletion.

Don't just show up. Think about *how* you'll show up. Then do what matters most—with your full presence and focus.

Assess where your energy flows each day. Are you giving your best to what truly moves the needle in your life? Are you nurturing relationships, goals, and habits that align with your highest self? Conserve energy by stepping away from what drains you and reinvesting that energy into what empowers you.

Are you spending your energy wisely or wasting it without return?

WHERE ROOTS GROW DEEP

The deepest roots grow where they are given adequate space.

The strongest connections don't flourish in constant closeness. Much like plant roots need room to reach down deep into the soil, the healthiest relationships grow stronger when space is given for trust to be established. Each person in a relationship brings their own previous journey, their own inner spark, their own story. Together, these two people can create something more beautiful than either could alone.

Love isn't about merging into one identity. It's about choosing to grow side by side, intertwined but not entangled. It's about knowing when to move closer with your presence and when to step back with trust. Real love allows space, not as distance but as sacred ground where individuality can thrive.

It sounds counterintuitive, but when you loosen your grip, instead of losing connection, you deepen it. When you say, "I trust you to become your true self, and I choose you still," love doesn't shrink but instead expands and grows into something beautiful.

Let your relationships breathe. Ask yourself: *Am I making space for others—and for myself—to grow, shine, and return freely?* Loosen the grip. Trust the dance.

What small step—either closer or farther—might bring more harmony, freedom, or depth into your relationships?

AUGUST

AUGUST 1

THE HUNGER BENEATH THE CRAVING

Emotional eating isn't really about food—
it's about filling something deeper
that your heart might be missing.

Many of us confuse consumption for comfort. Emotional eating often ramps up when something inside us feels hurt, unmet, or unresolved. Food, alcohol, endless scrolling, shopping, marathon-watching shows—whatever the outlet—becomes a stand-in for connection, peace, control, and healing.

In these moments, your hunger isn't for that bag of chips or pint of ice cream. It's for something much deeper inside your heart. When we slow down and truly listen—to our bodies and our minds and our hearts—we may find that what we're truly craving is to be heard, to be held, to be healed.

Reaching this place of awareness doesn't invite shame or restriction. Instead, if you've had this realization, approach it with curiosity and compassion. See it as an invitation to reconnect with yourself and respond with healing.

When you feel the pull to eat in response to emotion, take notice without judgment. Breathe. Ask yourself: *What do I actually need right now?* Instead of reaching for whatever comfort food, tend to that deeper need. You may find that the nourishment you're looking for has nothing to do with food.

How can you feed and nourish the truly hungry part of you in a way that actually heals?

BELIEVE BEYOND LIMITS

The biggest transformations come when we find the courage to believe beyond what we've been told.

Many of our limitations weren't born within us; they were passed down. Shaped by family, culture, or society, these beliefs often feel like truth, even when they don't actually reflect who we are or who we're becoming. We're told what success looks like, how to belong, what makes us worthy. But at some point, a quiet voice begins to ask: *Whose belief is this?*

That moment of questioning is the beginning of freedom. Because when we start to listen to what feels true within us—not what we were told—we begin to rewrite our stories.

Transformation doesn't require proving anyone wrong. It simply means we choose to trust ourselves enough to imagine a future that is more aligned, more authentic. Real change starts when we stop inheriting limits and start defining our own.

What belief have you been carrying around without ever challenging it? Today, pause and ask: *Does this still serve me? Is this really mine?* The courage to believe beyond outdated stories is the doorway to true growth. Choose a belief that uplifts and reflects who you truly are—not who you were told to be.

What new belief are you ready to claim as your own?

WHEN THE TIDE TURNS

The tide will turn. Patience holds more power than force, and time reveals what effort alone cannot.

We often believe that success comes only to those who push the hardest, move the fastest, or hustle the longest. But some of the greatest transformations don't come through force at all. They arrive through quiet persistence and deep trust. Patience isn't passive. It's a powerful form of discipline. It's the steady hand that keeps showing up even when there's no adoring crowd, no progress to post, no guarantee of results.

There are times in life when it feels like you're doing everything right—pouring in time, energy, and heart—and yet nothing seems to change. That's when our faith is tested. And that's when character is built. Because real growth often happens in the unseen. Beneath the surface. Beyond the timeline we imagined. And when the tide finally does turn, it's not by chance—it's because you held your ground when everything in you wanted to run.

If you're in a season of waiting, don't rush it. Stay rooted. Stay ready. You're not being overlooked; you're being prepared. The tide always turns, but only when you're patient enough to wait.

What part of your journey is calling for trust over urgency right now?

THE ART WITHIN THE STORM

Anxiety and creativity can be two sides of the same coin—one fuels the storm; the other turns it into art.

Anxiety can feel overwhelming—loud, consuming, impossible to control. It can arrive suddenly or simmer quietly beneath the surface. For many, the instinct is to fight, suppress, or avoid it.

But at its core, anxiety is energy—powerful, urgent, and deeply human. What if instead of resisting it, we learned to work *with* our anxiety? Rather than letting the anxiety take over, what if that restless energy were channeled into something creative such as writing, movement, music, or mindful expression? Although not a cure, mindfully engaging with your anxiety is a wonderful tool to help shift its hold on you. Over time, you may find a rhythm in how you respond to it. While anxiety may not fully disappear—and for some, professional support or treatment is essential—mindful practices can help. They can turn anxiety into insight, into art, into healing.

When your anxiety rears its head, pause and ask yourself: *What can I create with this?* Let your storm speak—not through panic but through purpose. Journal your thoughts. Paint your feelings. Dance through your tension. Creativity won't erase the storm, but it will give it form. And in that form, you can find freedom.

What storm within you is ready to be transformed into art?

AUGUST 5

ANSWERING COURAGE'S CALL

True courage knows when to rise, when to let go, and when to soar.

At one time or another, we've all bought into the belief that being courageous means never backing down and always pushing forward, even when the path clearly leads nowhere. But courage is far more nuanced. Courage isn't simply about persistence, pushing through obstacles, fighting against the headwinds, dusting yourself off again. Courage is actually deeply intertwined with wisdom.

Sometimes, the bravest step is to face a challenge head-on. Other times, it takes even more strength to let go of something that no longer serves you. True courage adapts rather than holding to a rigid set of standards. Being courageous doesn't mean you're always fighting. Instead, you discern which battles are worth your energy and when it's time to trust yourself and take flight—and then let yourself soar.

Pause and ask yourself: *What situation in my life is asking for a different kind of courage? Is it time to act? Or to finally let something go? Or to trust myself enough to soar?* Real courage aligns with truth. When you listen to your wisdom, the next step will become clear.

Where is courage calling you today? How will you answer with wisdom?

THE REALITY OF FEELING

Your emotions deserve care, even if they're invisible to others.

What you feel—every emotion, big or small—is real. Whether that feeling is rooted in fact or shaped by perception, your pain matters. So does your love. A fear, a loss, a longing—these feelings don't need outside validation to hold weight.

You may question your emotions, downplay your experiences, or tell yourself, *It wasn't that serious.* But the truth is, if a situation touched your heart or maybe even broke it, those feelings deserve attention and compassion. When you honor what you feel—without judgment or shame—you make space for healing. And you make space for wholeness.

Treat your inner world with the compassion it's been quietly asking for. You're not being dramatic. You're being human.

Offer compassion first—whether to yourself or to someone else. Don't dismiss pain simply because it doesn't make sense to you. Don't withhold love because you're unsure if it will be returned. Meet each emotion with presence and dignity. Healing will begin, and love will expand.

What would change in your life if you treated every emotion—yours and others'—as worthy of care?

ON THE OTHER SIDE OF FEAR

Happiness begins where fear ends.

Fear, more than any external obstacle, is often what holds us back from fully stepping into joy. Fear shows up in subtle ways—hesitation, perfectionism, self-doubt. It whispers, "What if you fail?" or "What if you're not enough?" We've all heard those voices. But we've also had moments when we pushed past them—when we took just one small step beyond the fear.

On the other side of fear isn't chaos, failure, or rejection; it's clarity, growth, and even joy. When we no longer allow fear to take the lead, joy finally has the space to rise. The most powerful shifts in life don't come from eliminating fear but from choosing to act in spite of it. And in making that choice—again and again—we reclaim freedom, peace, and a sense of purpose.

Courage isn't about having no fear; it's about trusting that something greater is waiting on the other side.

> What fear keeps tugging at your sleeve, keeping you from focusing on what you really want? Name it. Then take one step beyond that fear. You don't need to take a leap, just a step. Each step across that invisible line will move you closer to joy.

What happiness is waiting for you on the other side of fear?

EMBRACE THE JOURNEY

Being a champion means embracing the journey with gratitude, learning and celebrating along the way.

Real strength isn't found in perfection or nonstop progress. Real strength is found in the willingness to keep showing up, especially when things are hard. Gratitude can be an anchor in that process. Gratitude shifts our focus, helping us to see that even setbacks carry lessons, that slow steps are still steps forward.

Every stumble met with perseverance builds resilience.

Every small win reinforces momentum.

Viewing all of this through a lens of gratitude matters deeply—especially in a world that often pushes for perfection and speed. Life isn't a sprint. And there will be setbacks. But when we meet our journey with gratitude, patience, and curiosity, we create space for lasting growth.

Reflect today on how far you've come. Celebrate something you've learned, a challenge you've overcome, or a moment when you chose to keep going. No victory is too small. Whether you're facing uncertainty or navigating change, embrace gratitude for every moment that has taught you, moved you forward, or helped you persist.

In what ways can you honor your journey with compassion, courage, and gratitude?

TAKE THE WHEEL

The moment you realize you're not bound by your programming is the moment you take the wheel of your life.

We've all been shaped by our pasts—by habits, wounds, culture, and stories we didn't choose. But here's the truth: We're not stuck with the past. Our conditioning may explain us, but it doesn't define us. The patterns we have followed aren't permanent; they're just familiar. And familiarity isn't freedom.

Real freedom begins the moment you stop running on autopilot and start asking better questions. You're not a passenger in your own life. And the road isn't your master. You have the power to interrupt the cycle, redraw the map, and steer in a new direction.

The beliefs that once protected you might now be limiting you. But when you become aware of them—when you choose with intention rather than react out of habit—you take the wheel, and your course begins to change.

Pause and ask yourself: *What belief or behavior am I still letting drive my life?* Challenge that belief. Question it. Choose differently. The road doesn't determine your destination—you do.

What would your life look like if you stopped reacting and instead started driving with intention?

HEALING TOGETHER

In the warmth of genuine connection, we find the strength to overcome our deepest struggles.

The middle of hardship and unrelenting pain can feel like the loneliest place in the world. Deep pain often convinces us that we have to face it alone, that we must keep pushing through in silence, that no one will ever understand what we're going through.

But healing rarely begins in isolation. Often, the presence of another can help initiate healing. We're not talking about the people who try to fix us or react with judgment but rather the ones who sit with us in our darkness, who ask with care, who listen without judgment, who truly see us when we feel most invisible. Their empathy becomes a bridge—from isolation to belonging, from shame to hope.

True healing doesn't come from pretending to be strong. It comes from allowing ourselves to be vulnerable—to be seen, heard, and supported exactly as we are. That's where the real strength begins.

If you or someone you love is hurting, remember: No one has to face their pain alone. Healing starts with connection. Reach out. Let someone in. Be there. Together, we heal.

Who in your life needs your presence today? Are you letting them in when you need it most?

CHANGE FROM THE ROOT

The only way to truly change a behavior is to get to the root—the subconscious mind.

It's easy to assume that willpower alone is enough to help us change. You make a plan; you commit to try harder. And for a while, it works. But eventually, old patterns creep back in. That's because real change doesn't start with surface changes. It starts at the root—deep within the subconscious mind, where your beliefs, fears, and emotional habits live.

The subconscious is like soil. If the ground is filled with outdated beliefs or unresolved wounds, no amount of surface pruning will create lasting growth. True transformation requires looking inward with curiosity, not criticism. Ask yourself: *Why do I keep repeating this behavior? What story am I still living? Is my outside environment conducive to my health and well-being?*

The answers are there—beneath the noise, beneath the behavior—waiting to be seen, heard, and then rewritten. When you shift the story at the root, much of the behavior will change effortlessly.

Before you push harder, pause and listen for a moment. Journal, meditate, or reflect: *What belief is driving my action? What fear is shaping my choices?* Start from within, and the change will follow.

What belief might be silently shaping your behavior? Are you ready to rewrite that belief?

THE FOUR STEPS TO JOY

There are four steps to a joyful life—think well, eat well, act well, and most of all, be well.

Many people try to chase joy, hoping if they take this next adventure or acquire the next big thing, true happiness will finally be theirs. But joy isn't something you can capture. Joy is something you build. And often the building project starts with simple, intentional steps. When your thoughts are grounded, your meals are nourishing, your actions are purposeful, and your self-care nonnegotiable, things will begin to shift. Even your sleep will become more restful because your body and mind are no longer at war.

Think of joy as a rhythm—a rhythm you create by how you live. When you think well, you quiet the noise. When you eat well, you fuel your energy. When you act well, you walk in alignment. And when you *be* well—when you honor your needs and inner peace—you begin to glow from the inside out.

Take a moment to assess: *Which of these four areas is calling for my attention today—my mind, my health, my actions, or my intention?* Start small. Joy is built breath by breath, habit by habit.

Which of the four steps will you focus on first, and how will it shift your day?

AUGUST 13

THE KINDNESS WITHIN

No one can offer you more kindness than the kindness you give yourself.

Your relationship with yourself shapes every other part of your life. When your self-talk is critical, demanding, or unkind, it doesn't stay inside—it colors how you see the world, how you interact with others, and how you show up in the world. But when you practice kindness within—when you speak to yourself gently, give yourself grace, and honor your limits—everything begins to shift.

Kindness softens our sharp edges. It helps us breathe more deeply, act more intentionally, and connect with others from a place of wholeness. And kind self-talk isn't indulgent or selfish. It's essential, and it's an exercise in coming into alignment. The more you meet yourself with compassion, the more capacity you have to extend that compassion outward.

> Pause and notice the way you speak to yourself. Is it encouraging or critical? Uplifting or undermining? Work to begin shifting that inner voice toward kindness—not as a luxury but as an essential.

How can you offer yourself more kindness today? How might it change the way you show up in the world?

THE ROLE THAT FITS

Some lead, some follow. Both are important. The real question is which path aligns with your purpose.

Society often glorifies leadership, painting it as the most desirable role. What are we doing if we're not working our way up the ladder? But not everyone is meant to lead, and following isn't a weakness.

Greatness is found in self-awareness, in the wisdom to know when to step forward and when to support from behind. Without those willing to follow with intention, no vision could ever come to life. Without those ready to lead with purpose, there would be no direction. Choosing the right role for yourself isn't about status or recognition but about alignment. Are you leading from a place of clarity, service, and authenticity—or a desire for power? Are you following with belief and alignment—or out of fear, doubt, or a desire to please?

When we step into roles that reflect our true values—not what others might assign to us—we will discover ease, flow, and meaning.

In the different areas of your life, are you stepping into the roles that serve your highest purpose, or are you wearing titles that no longer fit? Honor where you truly thrive.

What role—leader or supporter—feels most aligned with your purpose right now? Are you brave enough to fully embrace it?

THE VOLUME OF SILENCE

Sometimes silence speaks the loudest—
if you're willing to truly listen.

In a world that prizes quick answers and constant noise, silence can feel uncomfortable, even threatening. But silence isn't empty—it's full of signals, insights, and emotional truths we often miss in the rush to respond or resolve problems. Some of the most powerful moments in life aren't filled with words but with presence. A quiet pause can speak louder than a long explanation. A moment of stillness can surface emotions we've buried or bring the clarity we didn't know we were searching for.

Silence isn't the absence of connection—it's often where the deepest connection begins. It gives you the space to process, to reflect, and to hear completely—yourself and others. When you learn to embrace it, silence becomes not just a pause but a powerful part of your voice.

The next time silence shows up, don't be so quick to fill it. Let it breathe. Whether in a conversation or in your own thoughts, give yourself permission to pause. Listen not just to what's being said but to what's not. In that space between words, wisdom, truth, and healing are waiting to be heard.

Where in your life do you need to listen more deeply? Could silence be the voice trying to reach you?

SIDE BY SIDE

True love is two people standing side by side, looking out on the same horizon.

Many of us think of love as getting lost in one another. But real love is about finding a shared path and walking it together. Constantly facing each other may look romantic, but over time it can lead to stagnation or unmet expectations. True connection is built when two people stand side by side—fully themselves, yet deeply united—looking toward something greater than either could reach alone.

When you share a horizon, love becomes a journey. It honors both independence and interdependence. It's not about agreeing on everything—it's about choosing to move in the same direction, even through the inevitable twists and turns of life. Side by side is where encouragement flows. It's where presence is quiet but powerful, where growth is supported, not stifled.

Think about the relationships that matter most to you. Are you walking together, or are you simply facing each other? Reconnect today, not just emotionally but also directionally. Clarify your shared goals, values, and purpose. Then step forward—together—with intention and love. That's where the bond deepens. That's where love lives and thrives.

Who is standing beside you, and what shared horizon are you walking toward?

LETTING GO OF OUTCOMES

Take aim with intention, and let go of the outcome.

Think about an archer. She draws the bow with full presence, focused on the target. And once she has released the arrow, the outcome is no longer in her control. Like the archer, we must aim with clarity, discipline, and heart—and then release the outcome, knowing it's not ultimately ours to control. In a world where success is so often defined by results, it's how we show up—focusing on effort over outcome—that determines our success.

Letting go doesn't mean giving up—it means trusting that your effort, rooted in intention, is enough. That's where peace lives. That's where growth happens. The arrow lands where it may, but the real transformation occurs in the strength it took to release it without fear or expectation. There is freedom to be found in focusing our attention on the process, not the result.

Today, focus on the process. Set your intention, take your best shot, and release any attachment to what follows. Show up with excellence rather than expectation. Trust that your growth is unfolding even if the target seems out of sight.

In what areas do you need to surrender the outcome and seek freedom in effort alone?

FROM LIMIT TO LAUNCHPAD

Today's limit is tomorrow's breakthrough.

What feels like a barrier today may be the very thing that fuels your transformation tomorrow. Limits aren't meant to confine you; they're meant to call you higher. Often, the moments that stretch you the most are the ones that result in the most growth and transformation.

A challenge can seem overwhelming when we're in the middle of it, but over time, those same struggles become proof of our strength. Limits are temporary. They shift when we do. Growth begins the moment we quit seeing obstacles as stop signs and start seeing them as stepping stones.

Each time you reach your edge and choose to keep going—one small step, one brave decision at a time—you begin to expand what's possible for you.

Take an honest look at what you've labeled as a limit in your life. Is it truly immovable, or is it waiting for you to challenge it? Lean into the discomfort. Approach it with consistency and self-belief. You don't have to break through overnight. Just keep pushing, keep growing. Today's ceiling can become tomorrow's floor.

What personal limit are you ready to challenge? How will you begin expanding beyond it?

THE FLY ON THE WINDOWPANE

We often fight the same barrier over and over, unaware that freedom lies in simply turning around.

We've all spent valuable time pressing hard against something that just wouldn't give—a goal, a belief, a relationship. We told ourselves that if we tried harder and pushed more, we would break through. But sometimes what kept us stuck wasn't a lack of effort but a lack of perspective. Like a fly banging itself against a windowpane, we might have been so focused on what was in front of us that we missed the clear path just behind us. But freedom doesn't always require struggle.

Sometimes, freedom is found in reflection. The breakthrough comes when you pause, step back, and ask: *Is the way I'm trying truly the only way?* Often, the barrier isn't blocking you—it's redirecting you. And what feels like resistance may simply be a sign to turn around and choose a new path.

If you're feeling stuck, don't push harder. Instead, look wider. Step back. Reevaluate. Let go of the need to force your way through, and trust the power of shifting direction. Your next move might not be forward. It could be a pivot that sets you free.

What are you still pushing through that may simply require a change in perspective?

INNER HYGIENE

Movement and meditation are like a shower for the inner self, cleansing and revitalizing us from within.

Hygiene for our outer physical bodies is instinctive—showering, grooming, dressing for the world. But what about our insides? Exercise and meditation aren't just wellness practices; they're inner hygiene.

Mindfulness and movement clear the clutter, drown out the noise, and flush out the tension we carry unconsciously. They cleanse us from within, leaving us grounded, focused, and fully alive. Exercise moves energy. It sweeps away stagnation and rewires our stress response. Meditation quiets the chaos, bringing us back to center. Together, they're an internal shower, rinsing off mental residue, recalibrating perspective, and anchoring us in the now.

You don't need to escape to the mountains to feel renewed. Simple acts—a quiet walk, deep breaths, stretching with intention—can strip away the weight of daily stress and restore your inner clarity. These aren't luxuries. They're maintenance. And they're how you return home to yourself, every single day.

Focus on your inner hygiene today. Give your soul a rinse. Move your body. Quiet your mind. Don't wait for overwhelm to take hold. Prevent it by cleaning out the chaos before it builds.

How can you make space today for five minutes of inner hygiene? What would that look like for you?

RISING BEYOND THE STORM

It's your choice whether to remain in
the rain or walk into the sun.

You didn't choose the storm. None of us do. But you do get to choose your next step. Life hits hard—unexpected loss, heartbreak, disappointment, instability. The rain may pour, but you don't have to stay soaked. This storm doesn't define who you are—or who you will become.

Strength isn't about avoiding the storm—it's about learning how to stand in the rain without letting it drown your spirit. Every moment you spend waiting for perfect conditions is a moment you could be growing and rising—and preparing for the next storm. You don't need to have everything figured out or know what's coming next. You just need to decide that your story doesn't end with the storm.

Breakthroughs don't come in dramatic flashes but in quiet choices to keep going. Courage and perseverance are built in those subtle moments when no one is watching but everything within you is changing.

Take a breath. Feel the ground beneath your feet. Then take one step forward, no matter how small. You cannot control what has already happened, but you hold the power to choose what happens next.

What's one storm you've survived? What's one way you can rise from it today?

AWARENESS BRINGS FREEDOM

What you recognize, you can master. What you ignore will master you. True freedom begins with awareness.

Awareness is the starting point of any real transformation, bringing unconscious patterns to light—those silent influences that shape our behaviors, choices, and emotions. When we ignore what's happening beneath the surface, those forces are allowed to run the show. But when we become aware of those patterns, even just a little, we create space for change.

Some of the most powerful shifts in our lives don't come simply from effort or forcing a change externally but from taking the time to *notice* what is happening so we can move forward in a mindful manner. This can look like noticing fear disguising itself as logic, or burnout whispering in the background as productivity, or a belief you have accepted for years no longer serving you. The simple act of awareness can become the turning point for a life of freedom.

Do you have a pattern, habit, or thought that keeps repeating? Don't rush to fix it; just acknowledge it. Awareness alone softens resistance and opens the door to clarity. Observed without judgment, what once controlled you becomes the very place you begin to find freedom.

Name an ignored thought or behavior that deserves your awareness today. How will you pause and give it attention?

WRITE YOUR OWN STORY

Don't settle for being a character in someone else's story. Instead, write your own story.

A time may come when you realize you've been living according to someone else's script, doing what is expected, following storylines others outlined, and measuring success by standards that were never truly yours.

Falling into a role someone else has written for you can happen quietly, almost invisibly. But once you realize your values, dreams, and voice don't line up with that role, you're able to start writing new scenes, to become the protagonist rather than a supporting character. When you start asking, *What really matters to me?* and have the courage to act on it, the plot for your life can change entirely.

Taking ownership of your story means picking up the pen—and writing a life that finally feels like *yours*.

Are you the author of your life or a character in someone else's plot? Reflect on where you've been letting others write your script. And then set one goal that reflects your truth—one *no* that honors your boundaries, one step in the direction of your dream. Reclaim the narrative. This is your story—and the world is waiting to read it.

What will your next chapter be, and will you be the one writing it?

CULTIVATING CONNECTION

Waiting for relationships to grow is like expecting a garden to flourish without watering it.

Connection doesn't happen by accident. Connection grows where it is cared for. Whether it's with a partner, a friend, a colleague, or even a stranger, meaningful relationships require presence, care, and intention. Much like a garden, they need planting, watering, and sunlight to grow.

Building connection isn't about grand gestures. Connection grows out of consistency. A thoughtful message, an open ear, a genuine smile—these small, deliberate efforts build trust and intimacy over time. When we expect closeness without investing time and energy, we set ourselves up for disappointment. But when we actively nurture our relationships, they begin to thrive, providing us with a deeper sense of belonging and mutual support.

Your intentional actions are the water that makes connection thrive.

Take a moment to reflect on how you're showing up in your relationships. Are you waiting for connection to magically appear, or are you planting the seeds daily? Choose to water what matters. Reach out. Listen. Be present. Even a small act of care can create powerful ripples.

Which relationship in your life—personal or professional—could grow stronger if you chose to nurture it more intentionally?

AUGUST 25

WORTHY OF THE WIN

If you want to win, you must believe you're worthy. Self-worth is the foundation of every lasting success.

You can train harder, plan smarter, and outwork everyone around you, but if deep down you don't believe you're worthy of the win, something inside will always hold you back. Quiet doubts will chip away at your potential, no matter how much effort you give. And missing out on the win won't be because of a lack of talent—it'll come from a lack of belief.

Self-worth isn't arrogance. It's a deep and grounded knowing. It's the quiet confidence of knowing you belong, even when no one's clapping. When you stand in that knowledge, you lead with presence, speak with truth, and act with purpose. You stop chasing approval and start owning your space. That kind of alignment creates consistency, courage, and a calm strength that others can feel—because instead of performing, you're *becoming*.

Don't just chase goals. Check your beliefs. Strengthen your self-worth like a muscle. When you know you're enough, the world will start feeling less like something you need to conquer and more like something you're ready to claim.

Do you believe you're worthy of the success you're working toward? Why or why not?

THE WIN IS IN THE WORK

The process matters more than the win because that's where you learn, grow, and discover yourself.

It's easy to become obsessed with outcomes. We chase the victory, the recognition, the final result. But in doing so, we risk missing the most valuable part of the journey—the work itself. The early mornings, the setbacks, the moments no one sees are where your character is being forged. You're facing your fears, refining your discipline, and discovering the grit that lives within you.

True growth doesn't happen suddenly once you cross the finish line. Every step you take toward the finish line is a victory. Wins are fleeting, but the lessons and strength you gain along the way stay with you. And ironically, when you commit to the process—fully and consistently—the outcomes often take care of themselves.

Winning isn't just about reaching the top. It's about who you become during the climb. That's the victory that lasts.

Refocus your energy on the effort, not the end goal. Be present for the process, and give yourself credit for every step forward.

What would shift in your life if you focused less on "winning" and more on how you show up each day to do the work?

HEALING THROUGH TRUTH

Sometimes simply speaking your truth brings healing. In sharing, we find connection and strength.

A quiet kind of pain can take root and grow in silence. We carry this pain alone, convinced that no one else would understand. But when we speak our truth, something shifts. It's about more than being heard. It's about being *seen*—and being seen changes everything.

Your truth doesn't have to be perfect, polished, or profound. It just has to be *yours*. In naming whatever is real and true for you, you reclaim your power from the lie that has held you back. Opening up about your truth gives shape to emotion, brings clarity to confusion, and shines light on the places where shame once tried to hide. When you speak up, you give others permission to do the same. Truth-telling is contagious. It dissolves isolation and connects us in our shared humanity.

So choose healing today. Instead of pretending to be fine, allow yourself to say what is true for you—even if you say it softly.

Share one truth today—with someone you trust or even just with yourself. Let it land without apology or explanation. Healing begins in honesty.

What part of your story have you kept quiet? How might your heart lighten or your connection with others deepen if you said it out loud?

AN INVITATION TO GROW

The ego resists correction, not because it knows best but because it fears being seen without its armor.

Growth rarely announces itself with comfort. It often arrives wearing the mask of discomfort—the sting of critique, harsh truths, or confrontation. In those moments, the ego rarely sees opportunity; it sees threat, rushing to defend, deflect, and deny, all to protect the image we've built.

Real transformation begins when we resist the urge to look away when someone or some difficult experience holds up a mirror. Instead of turning from what we may not want to see, we must choose to lean in closer. Correction doesn't diminish us; it refines us. Being wrong isn't weakness; it's an invitation to grow. The need to always be right is a trap. But being willing to learn with humility opens up a path toward real growth.

When we let humility lead, wisdom follows. With it comes clarity, resilience, and a freedom far greater than perfection could ever promise.

The next time feedback finds you, instead of armoring up, try opening up. Ask yourself: *Is this resistance protecting me, or is it preventing me from growing?* Let curiosity lead. Let truth instruct. Release the need to be right so you can rise into what's possible.

Who could you become if you were brave enough to listen fully?

THE QUESTIONS THAT GUIDE YOU

Who am I? and *Why am I here?* aren't questions to solve, but doors to walk through.

Some questions aren't meant to be answered. They're meant to be lived. *Who am I?* and *Why am I here?* aren't riddles to decode or problems to fix. They're invitations. Openings. Portals into something deeper than certainty. Gateways to purpose, presence, and becoming.

You may not always have the words, but your life speaks for you. With every choice, every act of courage, every time you listen to what feels aligned, you step further into who you truly are. You don't find your purpose all at once—it unfolds little by little. Purpose reveals itself when you show up, when you listen, when you move even when you're unsure.

Trying to figure it all out at once can keep you stuck. But asking questions as you go keeps you moving toward exactly where you need to be.

Let the questions stay open. Walk through them. Live in them. And let each brave step forward show you more than answers ever could.

What's one step you can take today—not to solve your purpose, but to walk deeper into it?

THE WISDOM OF INTUITION

If something excites you, lean in. But if an idea causes your gut to tighten, your intuition is speaking.

We're trained to trust data, logic, and rationale, but another factor often speaks first and truest: *intuition*. This voice doesn't appear on spreadsheets or analysis reports. Intuition shows itself as a subtle knowing, a feeling, a signal deep within your body. Sometimes it's a lightness pulling you forward. Sometimes it's a tension begging you to stop.

This isn't superstition—it's a different kind of intelligence. Your nervous system has been gathering information for a long time, often long before your conscious mind catches on. Intuition is your body's way of whispering what your soul already knows. You're not ignoring facts; you're integrating them with an inner wisdom that's always been there.

Your most aligned decisions happen when your mind understands what your body is already sensing. The challenge is getting quiet enough to hear it—and brave enough to trust it.

Before you act, pause and ask yourself: *Does the decision I'm about to make open something in me or close something down?* Then listen—with your whole being. When you tune in to your intuition, you don't just react—you respond with grounded clarity.

What big decision are you facing right now, and what does your body already know about it?

THE FORWARD MOTION OF INNOVATION

Innovation isn't about starting from scratch—
it's about finding new ways forward.

We often think innovation means starting from scratch, creating something the world has never seen. But true innovation often begins with a shift in perspective. It's not always about *invention* but rather about *insight*. Sometimes, the most meaningful progress comes from reimagining what already exists, seeing the familiar through a new lens, and asking: *How can this serve me—and others—more deeply?*

Growth isn't always about tearing down the old and replacing it with something new but instead evolving what already exists. When we embrace the mind-set of innovation, creativity becomes accessible to all of us, inviting us to think differently, act boldly, and transform the ordinary into something extraordinary.

Rather than waiting for the perfect original idea, take stock of what's already in motion around you. Ask yourself: *What can I improve, refine, or reimagine?* Whether it's in your work, your wellness, or your relationships, innovation often begins by pointing something familiar in a bold, new direction.

What are you already working with that, by shifting your perspective, could become something extraordinary?

SEPTEMBER

A TURNING POINT IN DISGUISE

Quitting isn't an option—it's a distraction from success.

Every meaningful pursuit comes with challenges. Whether you're chasing a goal, nurturing a relationship, or working through a personal transformation, there will be moments when quitting is tempting. But what often seems like an end is actually a turning point in disguise.

Perseverance is what transforms difficulty into progress and effort into achievement. There is no straight line to success. Achieving a goal or reaching a destination demands consistency, patience, and the willingness to keep moving forward, even (and especially) when things get difficult or uncomfortable.

The people who grow most and reach the biggest goals aren't always the fastest or the strongest. They're the ones who *keep going* when others stop. Because they know that quitting doesn't remove the challenge, only the possibility of overcoming it. And you *can* overcome it if you view challenges as opportunities.

When obstacles show up, pause—but don't retreat. Ask yourself: *What am I working toward that's worth enduring discomfort for?* Progress is rarely dramatic. Most often, it's quiet, steady, and built on a repeated decision not to give up. Stay with the process. Stay with your vision. Success isn't found in ease but in endurance.

What part of your journey today is calling for one more step?

WHAT TRULY LASTS

Victory lasts for an instant, but what
got you there lasts forever.

That moment of triumph—crossing the finish line, sealing the deal, achieving the goal—feels electric. But then it's gone in a flash. The crowd quiets. The trophy gathers dust. And what we're left with isn't the win itself. What stays is the person we became along the way. The discipline it took to stay consistent. The resilience we built through failure. The quiet choices we made when no one was watching. That's the part that endures.

The process doesn't just get you there—it builds you. It shapes your mind-set, your strength, your integrity. And in those moments when motivation fades, that foundation becomes your fuel. The spotlight fades, but character remains. Victory is a snapshot. Your journey is the story. And that will stay with you long after the celebration ends.

Celebrate the wins, but don't overlook what made them possible. Honor your growth. Value your path. The outcome isn't what defines you. The work that prepared you to reach it speaks volumes about your true self.

Are you chasing the moment? Or are you cultivating character that can rise to the occasion, again and again?

PURPOSE GIVES REASON

If you have purpose, you have a reason to keep going.

Purpose isn't just an idea; purpose is fuel. It's the quiet fire that keeps you moving when everything else tells you to stop.

Life will challenge you. The path will twist. In many moments, exhaustion will whisper, "Why bother?" But when you're anchored in purpose, you always have an answer. Purpose gives meaning to the effort, to the discomfort, to the discipline. It transforms the mundane into the meaningful. You're no longer just working—you're building something that matters.

Purpose doesn't need to be grand or loud. It just needs to be *yours*. Whether it's caring for someone, mastering a craft, creating impact, or simply becoming the best version of yourself, that internal compass will keep you aligned when life gets heavy. Without this focus, even small setbacks will feel overwhelming. But with it, the tallest mountains are climbable.

Reignite your connection to what matters most. Say it out loud. Write it down. Carry it with you. When purpose leads, strength follows. When purpose is clear, progress is inevitable.

What is one purpose, big or small, that gives your life direction right now? Are you letting it lead the way?

YOUR UNIQUE PLACE IN THE WORLD

You may not see it yet, but there's a place in this world that only *you* can fill.

All of us at some point question our role, our value, where we truly belong. Maybe you feel like a puzzle piece that doesn't quite fit into the bigger picture. But you're not here to squeeze into someone else's design. You're meant to create your own masterpiece.

You carry a unique combination of gifts, struggles, dreams, and wisdom that no one else has. And that's not by accident. When you begin to trust what makes you uniquely *you*, even before it makes sense or your purpose fully reveals itself, something inside you will shift.

The path may not be clear, but your place on that path is real. Keep showing up. Keep believing. The world is waiting for what only you can bring.

If you've ever felt out of place, let that feeling be a sign. It could be how your calling is being revealed. Stay curious. Grow through uncertainty. You don't need to have all the answers in order to take the next step.

What part of you are you still holding back? What would it look like to offer it boldly to the world?

THE GIFT OF RECOGNITION

The greatest gift you can give another is sincere recognition for how they've touched your life.

In our fast-moving lives, it's easy to unintentionally overlook the quiet efforts of those around us. Yet what most people crave isn't more attention or praise. Most of us want to feel deeply seen and acknowledged.

True recognition goes beyond paying a compliment. What touches a person's spirit is an acknowledgment of their presence, intention, and the impact they make simply by being themselves. It's saying, "I noticed you," in a way that validates both their actions and their essence. Recognizing another individual's contributions can lift them far more than any material gift ever could.

Meaningful and intentional recognition creates connection, healing, and lasting encouragement through a single sentence. The gift of recognition reminds us that what we do—and who we are—truly matters.

Who in your life has shown up, supported you, or quietly made a difference? Offer them a heartfelt acknowledgment so they know they are seen and valued. Recognition isn't about ceremony but about sincerity.

Who will you recognize today? How might that acknowledgment change their day—or even their life?

THE DISAPPEARING BRIDGE

When "I" and "me" crowd out "us" and "we," the bridge of connection turns to rubble.

Relationships don't thrive on ego—they thrive on empathy. When communication becomes dominated by "I" and "me," the invisible bridge that connects two people begins to weaken. Individuality matters. But without the balance of mutual respect and collective thinking, connection falters.

The healthiest relationships are built on inclusion, not isolation. Cooperation, not competition. True connection means seeing beyond your own needs to recognize and value the needs of others. "Us" and "we" create space for trust, unity, and shared purpose. They transform conversations into collaboration and conflict into understanding.

When we operate from a place of self-interest, we may find ourselves standing on one side of a broken bridge—alone, unheard, and disconnected.

Pay attention to how you speak and act in your relationships. Are you building connection or creating distance? Begin shifting your language and intention. Use words that invite, include, and honor togetherness. Choose presence over pride. Because connection isn't about winning—it's about walking across the bridge together.

What bridge in your life needs rebuilding, and are you willing to meet in the middle?

THE POWER OF RISK

Risk may lead to failure or success, but refusing to take it ensures you'll experience neither.

Risk sits at the center of every meaningful breakthrough. Whether it's launching something new, speaking an important truth, or simply choosing a change for your life, risk always comes with uncertainty. But so does growth.

Playing it safe may feel comfortable, but comfort often leads to stagnation. What many of us truly fear isn't failure but regret. Because even failure teaches us. It builds resilience, sharpens our focus, and redirects us toward something better. But refusing to try? That teaches us nothing. It leaves us wondering, *What if?*

Not all risks are flashy. Sometimes they're quiet acts of courage—being vulnerable, taking a different path, betting on yourself. And when you move with intention, those small choices often lead to your most powerful transformations.

Think about a risk you've been avoiding. What's really stopping you—fear, comfort, or the illusion of certainty? Weigh the cost of staying still against the potential for growth. Your next step doesn't have to be perfect. The only regret you'll have is if you don't take it.

What risk are you finally ready to take, not despite your fear but because of what's possible beyond it?

WHEN *NOT* TO FOLLOW

The most powerful teachers often show us who we don't want to become.

Inspirational people cross our paths daily. But growth doesn't only come from those who inspire. Sometimes those who challenge, disappoint, or even hurt us are our most important teachers.

Life is generous with its teachers, but not all of them bring warmth, wisdom, or worth. Some serve as mirrors that, rather than reflecting our highest selves, instead reveal important boundaries. These individuals help refine our values and show us what we refuse to tolerate, who we won't become, and which paths we'll never walk again. They also bring us clarity about what integrity looks like and help uncover the kind of presence and ethics we want to offer the world. These lessons may sting in the moment, but they bring us face-to-face with our truest identity—not through imitation but through alignment with our values.

We don't always get to choose the messengers life brings us, but we do get to choose the message we carry forward.

When someone challenges your peace, don't react. Instead, reflect: *What is this situation revealing about who I'm becoming?* Not every person is worthy of emulating. Sometimes we must set a boundary and choose a different path.

What have your most difficult encounters or relationships taught you about who you're committed to becoming?

THE VOICE OF COMPASSION

Self-compassion means choosing a different voice—a voice of love, healing, and truth.

Sometimes the harshest things we say to ourselves don't actually originate from within. Instead, they're inherited echoes. Words others have spoken to us in anger, disappointment, or judgment can embed themselves so deeply that we mistake them for truth. Over time, these echoes shape an inner critic that grows louder than our own voice of reason.

Awareness offers a way out. We don't have to keep replaying those old scripts. We can choose a voice that reflects our growth, not our wounds. Self-compassion isn't weakness—it's the courageous act of rewriting the story. It means meeting our flaws with patience, our pain with gentleness, and our progress with celebration.

Pay attention to your self-talk today. Is it empowering or defeating? Understanding or judgmental? Encouraging or negative? Begin to replace every judgment with encouragement, every doubt with truth. Speak to yourself as you would speak to someone you love deeply. You are worthy of that same care and kindness.

How would it feel if your inner voice became your greatest ally instead of your harshest critic?

THE POWER OF SELF-TALK

The words you speak to yourself have the power to shape your reality.

One of the most powerful influences on our mind-set, performance, and emotional well-being is the way we speak to ourselves. That inner voice is always there—shaping how we show up, how we cope, how we grow. When it's kind, supportive, and rooted in belief, it gives us the strength to rise. But when that voice turns critical or doubtful, it becomes a weight that holds us back.

We tend to become what we repeatedly tell ourselves we are. Do you think you're lazy? You will be. That you'll never get it right? Wait for that to come true. That you're not worthy of love? Love will have a harder time finding you.

Our thoughts aren't just passing words; they're seeds. And whatever we plant, we eventually grow into. Choose your inner language with care. Speak to yourself as someone worth believing in—because you are.

When negativity shows up, don't judge it. Instead, redirect it. Affirm your strengths. Encourage your progress. Your internal words can be your greatest ally or your loudest enemy. Choose to be on your own side. When you believe in yourself, the world will reflect that belief right back.

What will you say to yourself today to move closer to the life you want?

THE SWEET REWARDS OF PATIENCE

The sweetest rewards come to those who understand the power of patience.

In a world that glorifies speed and instant results, patience can feel like falling behind. But in truth, patience is a quiet power we all have the capacity to cultivate. The most meaningful changes—healing, growth, love, purpose—don't happen overnight. They unfold slowly, shaped by consistency, setbacks, and grace.

Patience isn't about doing nothing. Patience is active trust. It's choosing to stay the course when progress is invisible. It's believing in your path even when the world pressures you to rush. More often than not, impatience is just fear in disguise—fear that whatever we're waiting for won't happen or that we're not enough without constant achievement. But patience speaks from a deeper place. It softly reminds us: *You're not behind; you're unfolding right on schedule.*

Lasting change takes time. And the moments that truly matter are worth the wait.

Look at an area of your life where you're craving quick results. Can you offer that situation more patience? More presence? Keep showing up, but release your need to rush. Trust that the timing of your growth, your healing, and your success is unfolding exactly as it should.

What reward are you willing to wait for because you know it's worth it?

THE ECHO OF ACTION

Action speaks louder than words—
and louder still than intention.

We often mistake good intentions for progress. We dream. We plan. We speak about what we'll do . . . someday. But intention without action is like a song never sung, a path never walked. It may echo with potential, but it leaves no imprint.

There's nothing wrong with vision. But only when vision is paired with movement does it begin to shape reality. The shift happens the moment we stop waiting for permission, perfection, or the "right time" and start taking that first, brave step, no matter how small.

The people who change their lives, who shape the world around them, don't just think or speak—they *do*. And even imperfect action carries more weight than the most polished intention left idle. Put actions, not intentions, to work in your life.

Ask yourself: *What intention have I held on to without taking any movement?* Today, close the gap between desire and decision. Make the call. Take the step. Begin. Let your action be the echo that inspires—not just within but far beyond.

What is one action you can take today to turn your silent intention into a living reality?

SEPTEMBER 13

YOU ARE THE AUTHOR OF YOUR LIFE

You are not the product of your history.
You are the author of your life.

You aren't defined by what happens to you. It may feel that way sometimes, but you are defined by what you do with what happens to you and what you choose next. Yes, your past shapes you, but it doesn't hold the pen. Whatever experiences, mistakes, and setbacks you encounter are pages, maybe even chapters, but they aren't the whole book of your life.

Too often, you might get stuck rereading old chapters, letting them dictate your self-worth or your potential. But the pen has always been in your hand. You get to choose how the story evolves. With every moment of awareness, every act of bravery, every step toward healing, you're writing the next line of your story—on your terms.

The most powerful stories aren't flawless from the start. The stories that move us are the ones where the protagonist rises up from something difficult, reclaims the narrative, and transforms pain into purpose.

Ask yourself: *What chapter of my life am I ready to begin writing?* Then take one bold step in that direction. You aren't a victim of your history. You are your life's author and editor.

If you saw yourself as the author of your story, what would you begin writing today?

THE DOORWAY TO UNDERSTANDING

Empathy begins where judgment ends.

It's easy to watch someone else's struggles and offer commentary. From the outside, a solution can seem simple, clear, even obvious. But life is rarely what we observe. Hidden layers tell a deeper story. And real understanding doesn't come from analysis or opinion but rather from presence. When we pause to consider what someone might be feeling, when we stop evaluating and start relating, when we listen rather than commenting, something powerful happens: Empathy enters the room.

Empathy doesn't require agreement. It doesn't demand justifying someone's actions or taking on their pain. It only asks that we acknowledge their humanity—that we see the person behind the behavior. In a world that's quick to judge and slow to listen, this kind of awareness is radical. It transforms criticism into compassion and turns conflict into connection.

We all want to be understood, not fixed or dismissed. And the fastest way to offer that gift to others is to ask, *What if that were me?*

The next time you feel the urge to judge or offer advice, ask yourself what that person might be carrying that you can't see. Let empathy guide your perspective and help you find understanding.

Where in your life could you replace judgment with empathy? What might that shift?

SEPTEMBER 15

THE WISDOM OF FLEXIBILITY

The true power of a plan is in having a Plan B.

Flexibility isn't weakness; it's wisdom in motion. You might start out with a clear vision, but when reality shifts—as it so often does—the ability to pivot is what will keep you moving forward. Clinging to one fixed outcome or path can lead to frustration and burnout. But when you're open to Plan B (or even Plan C), you can stay in the game. Instead of giving up, you adapt. And that's where your wisdom really shows.

Progress doesn't always follow a straight line, but with flexibility, you'll still arrive where you're meant to be. You learn to trust the journey, even when the destination moves or changes. And in that trust, you will gain resilience, creativity, and unstoppable momentum.

Take a look at your current goals. If Plan A doesn't work out, what's your next move? Don't wait for a crisis to force creative thinking. Build flexibility into your mind-set now. Life rewards those who bend but don't break. Your ability to adapt might just be your greatest advantage.

How will you strengthen your flexibility today—mentally, emotionally, or practically?

THE DEVOTION OF SEEING

Truly seeing someone—fully, wholly—
is the rarest form of devotion.

In a world of rapid scrolls, quick greetings, and distracted conversations, the act of truly seeing someone is revolutionary. To see is not just to look upon—it's to *be with.* It's holding space for someone's truth without fixing, judging, or rushing them through it. It's witnessing not just their words but the silence behind them.

To truly see another is to meet them where they are, not where we wish they were. When we commit to seeing another, we acknowledge the totality of their experience—the visible and the hidden—and we say, "I see you, and I'm staying." This kind of presence heals. It tells the person, "You matter." It builds safety, trust, and love without actually saying a word.

This level of devotion doesn't demand grand gestures. It simply asks you to be *here*, fully and sincerely. And in a world starving for connection, few gifts are more sacred.

Be the one who sees today. Pause. Listen beyond the surface. Look beyond the role someone plays and meet their humanity. Offer the kind of presence that doesn't try to force a solution and instead acts as a witness.

**Who in your life might be waiting—
hoping—to finally feel seen by you?**

PURSUE PEACE

Peace isn't found in the absence of noise. It's found in the presence of inner stillness.

Oftentimes we believe we'll experience peace when life finally quiets down. *As soon as I finish this big project, I'll catch my breath. Once the kids are off to school, we'll finally find time to reconnect with one another.* But peace is something we can embrace in the middle of the noise. Rather than silence after a storm, peace is the stillness we carry into that storm.

We don't have to escape the chaos to pursue peace. Life is busy. That's not likely to change. We choose peace by not letting that busyness enter our *inner* world. We pause before reacting. We observe without absorbing. We stay grounded when everything feels shaky.

Being at peace doesn't mean you don't care. It means you've learned to care *wisely,* without letting outside turbulence unsettle your inner compass. And the more you cultivate that stillness, the more it becomes your default and a mind-set you embody.

Make space for stillness today. Whether you slow down to breathe deeply, stop for a moment of silence, or take a walk without your phone, choose to return to yourself. Peace begins within, not after everything else ends.

What might change in your life if you chose to pursue peace instead of waiting for it?

LET REGRET BE YOUR TEACHER

We can learn from regret—and then we need to break free.

Regret tends to follow us like a lingering shadow, always tapping us on the shoulder. Maybe it's an opportunity you let slip away, words you couldn't take back, a mistake you wished you could undo. The weight of regret can feel heavy long after the incident has passed. It has a way of draining your energy and clouding your self-worth. But what would happen if you stopped seeing regret as a punishment and started viewing it as a teacher?

When we let regret teach us, it becomes a guide rather than an indictment. No amount of regret will undo what has already happened. But there's good news: The size of the stumble we took doesn't matter. We can always make peace with the pain and allow it to inform a better future. What happened then matters far less than the choice you make now.

Think of a regret you've been holding on to. Instead of replaying the pain, ask yourself: *What did this experience teach me?* Use that insight as fuel for growth rather than shame. You can't change the past, but you can choose how it shapes you.

What weight are you willing to leave behind, and what wisdom are you ready to carry forward?

THE POWER OF REASON

Shouting settles nothing. Only reason
and restraint lead to resolution.

In moments of tension, shouting may feel like a release, a way to assert control or direct another person's attention. But shouting or responding in anger almost aways leads to more division than resolution. When voices rise, ears close. And instead of solving the problem, we end up deepening the conflict.

True strength lies not in overpowering someone but in staying composed enough to communicate with clarity and calmness. Reason softens defenses. Restraint opens the door to listening. When we respond thoughtfully rather than react impulsively, we create the conditions for real understanding.

Your motivation shouldn't be about winning the argument; it should be about protecting the relationship. Choosing reason over reaction is the clearest expression of maturity and wisdom.

When a conflict starts to heat up, pause and allow yourself to feel the emotion. But don't let it dictate your next step. Ask yourself: *What outcome do I truly want here?* Then speak with intention. The power to defuse conflict is in your presence, your tone, and your willingness to listen.

What would it look like to lead with reason rather than reaction in your most difficult conversations?

TRUST THE CLOSED DOORS

Every closed door is guiding you closer
to the door you're meant to open.

There are times in life when something we deeply hoped for—an opportunity, a relationship, a dream—doesn't unfold the way we imagined it would. In those moments, it's easy to feel discouraged or even question our path. But what feels like a setback may actually be a form of protection or redirection.

Life often has a bigger picture in store—one that's preparing us for something more aligned with who we're becoming. You might not see it right away, but with time and reflection, your vision will become clearer. What doesn't work out often opens up space for something far more meaningful. Detours, delays, even rejections—they're not signs of failure. They're invitations to trust, grow, and realign with your truest path.

If you're facing a closed door, resist the urge to force it open. Instead, reflect on what that closed door might be teaching you or saving you from. Trust that not every denial is a loss. Some things simply aren't yours to carry forward. Stay open to a new path. The door meant for you will appear when you're ready for it.

What possibility might be waiting for you behind the next door if you're willing to move on from the last one?

BEYOND THE SKY

Your only limits are those you place on yourself.
Break those, and the sky is just the beginning.

Many of us believe our limitations are out there—too little time, not enough opportunity, no support. But when we look closer, we often find that the most impenetrable barriers aren't external at all. Our limitations come from within.

Fear of failure.

Fear of judgment.

Doubt dressed up as caution.

These invisible ceilings feel real because we've been carrying them for so long. But the moment we question those beliefs, something shifts. We realize that courage isn't the absence of fear; it's the willingness to move forward with fear still in our pocket. Every time we break through an internal wall, a new horizon appears. And suddenly, we see it clearly: Limitations cannot confine us if we're willing to break through the barriers we built within.

What belief or fear have you mistaken for truth? Name it. Question it. Then take one bold step beyond it—because your next chapter begins beyond the limits you've accepted.

What limit will you choose to go beyond today, and what might be possible on the other side?

FEAR DOESN'T DEFINE YOU

Silence fear and doubt in order to see your value and hold on to your self-worth.

Fear has a quiet way of slipping into the driver's seat of our lives. It doesn't always shout—often it whispers. It tells us we're not ready, not smart enough, not deserving. And when we listen too long, we begin to believe those stories. We begin to shrink in places where we were meant to rise. We begin to forget our value.

Here's the truth: Fear does not get to define you. The measure of your worth was never meant to be affected by the presence of doubt. Your worth is affirmed by your courage—your ability to keep showing up even when uncertainty looms. Every time you act in alignment with your values instead of your fears, you reclaim a part of yourself. You step forward. You grow.

Self-worth isn't a destination. It's a decision—one you make again and again, especially when fear tries to steer you off course. The more you practice believing in your value, the quieter fear becomes.

Take a breath and notice where fear may be influencing your decisions. Choose to lead with self-worth instead of fear. Speak truth to dispel your doubt, and step forward in courage.

Where in your life are you letting fear define your worth? What would change if you stopped?

THE POWER TO PIVOT

You have the power to let go of what isn't working and lean fully into what is.

There's strength in staying the course. Commitment is a deeply valued attribute. But there is also deep wisdom in knowing when to step onto a new path. Many of us believe that commitment means never turning back, never changing direction, even when whatever we're pursuing no longer aligns with who we're becoming. We cling to paths, patterns, people, and places out of fear—fear of judgment, failure, or the unknown.

But here's the truth: Pivoting isn't weak. Choosing to alter your course is a sign of true bravery. Rather than signaling failure, a pivot reveals that you listened to your body, your intuition, your truth. Whether it's a job, a relationship, a mind-set, or a habit, what once served you may no longer fit. And that's not a cue to push harder. It's a call to pause, breathe, adjust . . . and then step onto a new path.

The most aligned lives don't follow a straight line. Their trajectory is shaped by bold, honest turns.

What in your life feels misaligned? What is asking to be released? What is asking to be fully embraced? Trust yourself. One small pivot can redirect your entire future.

If today were your turning point, where would you choose to go from here?

THE PERSPECTIVE SHIFT

What you see as your prison may
actually be your launching pad.

Life has a way of disguising growth as struggle. What might feel like confinement—an unchanging situation, a personal setback, a challenge you didn't ask for—can often be the very ground on which transformation begins. The walls that seem to box you in might actually be the edges from which you learn to push off.

Your growth is less about circumstance and more about the mind-set you bring to that circumstance. When you reframe your struggle as preparation instead of punishment, prepare for a shift. Power begins with perspective. Change the way you see a struggle, and you will change the way you move through it—with courage, clarity, intention, and an unshakable belief that even *this* is part of becoming.

Take a fresh look at your current challenge. Instead of asking, *Why is this happening to me?* ask, *What is this preparing me for?* Stand with strength, shift your perspective, and let your limitations fuel your rise.

How might your current struggle be shaping your next breakthrough?

THE FRAGILE MASTERPIECE

A habit is a fragile masterpiece—built with patience, broken in a blink.

Habits aren't just routines. They're reflections of who you're becoming. It takes time, care, and repetition to shape them. One choice at a time, you lay a foundation. But even the strongest habits can crack under pressure, fatigue, or old patterns. This doesn't make you a failure—it makes you human.

Growth isn't a straight line. It's a dance between progress and pause, discipline and distraction. It doesn't matter how many times you fall. It only matters that you get back up. Maybe you skipped the gym for a week, slipped into late-night scrolling, or let your journal collect dust. These slip-ups don't erase your progress—they're simply reminders to begin again. Each restart strengthens resilience. Each moment of recommitment is proof you're still in the game.

The beauty of a habit lies in its fragility. It teaches you presence. It humbles you. It reminds you mastery isn't about never breaking but about how quickly you can begin again.

Treat your habits like art—worth protecting, worth returning to again and again. Be gentle with your process. You're not failing when you falter. You're growing every time you recommit.

When you slip, do you shame yourself or do you choose to rebuild with compassion and clarity?

STRIKING THE BALANCE

Nutrition and movement work hand in hand. What you feed your body fuels your outcomes.

It's easy to focus on one pillar of well-being while unintentionally neglecting another. Many people find themselves showing up consistently for their workouts or daily movement—whether it's hitting the gym, going for walks, or taking time to stretch—yet they struggle to see or feel the progress they're working so hard for. The missing link? *Nourishment.*

What we eat isn't just about satisfaction or addressing hunger. Mindful eating is about fueling and nourishing our body and mind for the very effort we're putting into becoming stronger, healthier, and more energized. True transformation happens when nutrition and movement are in sync.

When the fuel supports the function, the results are not only visible; they're also intrinsic—in our energy, our confidence, and our clarity.

Are your eating habits truly supporting your desire to feel better, move better, and live better? Start small. Choose foods that nourish, eat with intention, and focus on hydration. Perfection isn't the goal. You're looking to create alignment and intention in your choices. When your nutrition and movement are speaking the same language, your body will pay attention.

How would your life change if your fuel consistently matched your effort?

JUDGMENT AND THE MIRROR

We see in others what we refuse to see in ourselves.

It's so easy to judge. To point out flaws, critique behavior, or measure others by standards we ourselves struggle to meet. But unchecked judgment reveals more about the judge than the judged. It exposes insecurity masked as superiority and projection disguised as principle. Before we critique, we must reflect.

Are we truly better than the person we're judging, or are we choosing to remain blind to our own flaws? Have we mastered what we condemn? Or are we hiding behind comparison to avoid our own need for growth? The truth is, we all fall short. We all stumble, hesitate, repeat the same mistakes, and need grace. And when we approach a situation with reflection rather than reaction, we create space for understanding.

Judgment shuts down growth. Humility opens the door to growth—for others and for ourselves.

The next time you feel the urge to judge, pause and ask yourself: *Am I offering enlightenment or simply casting a shadow on someone else's struggle?* Turn the mirror inward. Growth begins with honest self-awareness—and so does compassion.

What personal struggle in others have you judged that may be alive and unspoken in you?

THE LOVE YOU GROW INTO

Each connection carries pieces of the past, shaping the love you're finally ready to see and hold.

Love rarely starts from scratch. The way you love now—the depth, the caution, the openness—was shaped by every connection that came before. Some past relationships taught you to set boundaries. Others cracked you open to vulnerability. Some reminded you of what you deserve. Others revealed what you'll never settle for again.

Every heartbreak and healing carved space for the kind of love you're now capable of receiving. That's not baggage—it's growth. You're not walking into new love empty-handed. You're bringing the wisdom of lived experience, the softness that comes from healing, and the clarity that only time can offer.

You aren't rewriting your story. And falling in love isn't the first chapter. You're continuing to write the book—with more awareness, more honesty, and more heart.

Embrace where you've been. Let your past shape you instead of hardening you. Show up for love with your eyes wide open and your heart willing. You're not starting over; you're arriving ready.

How has your past shaped the way you love today? Are you ready to love with all that you've learned?

THE FOUNDATION OF SOLUTIONS

Build an environment where solutions take root.

Problems are a part of life. But whether they linger or lead to transformation often depends on the environment we create, both internally and externally. When we focus solely on the issue—replaying it, analyzing it, or blaming others—we keep ourselves stuck in a loop.

But when we foster an environment grounded in curiosity, clarity, and calm, something powerful happens: Solutions begin to take root. This shift isn't about ignoring difficulties or rushing past real emotions. Instead, you're asking better questions, engaging in open dialogue, and creating space for answers to emerge. A solution-focused environment is one where fear doesn't dominate, criticism doesn't paralyze, and progress isn't dependent on perfection. It's one where frustration is turned into fuel and setbacks transform into stepping stones.

Whether in your home, your workplace, or your own mind, when you intentionally cultivate a space where growth is welcomed and forward motion is valued, you'll notice that even the most complex problems begin to unravel.

Today, reflect on the environment you're creating. Are you nurturing problems or cultivating solutions? Make a conscious shift toward clarity, collaboration, and action. That's where real change takes root.

How can you shift your environment to better support solutions?

LET THEM BECOME

Your kids are yours, but they are not you.
Let them be who they're meant to be.

As parents, we feel a responsibility not just to raise our children, but to *shape* them. We want to pass down what we know, protect them from hardships, and sometimes fulfill dreams we never chased. But in doing so, we cast a shadow where their light could shine.

Your child isn't your second chance. They're not your mirror or unfinished story. They are their own person, with their own rhythm and destiny. While your love should guide them, it should never confine them. The hardest part of parenting isn't holding on—it's letting go. Not of care or support, but expectations.

And if you're reading this not as a parent but as someone's child, take heart. Your parents' hopes may not always match your own. Their love may feel heavy with expectation, but you were never born to carry their story. You were born to write your own. Being allowed to become who we are is the purest love we can be offered.

If you're a parent, ask your child what they want—not what *you* want. We all deserve to grow beyond the blueprint we were handed.

Where might expectations—yours or someone else's—limit your freedom to grow into your true self?

OCTOBER

THE POWER OF THOUGHT

The more you linger on negative thoughts, the more power you give them to become your reality.

Your mind is a garden, and every thought is a seed. What you focus on, you feed. If you constantly water fear, doubt, worry, or regret, those feelings will grow, choking out confidence, joy, and potential. Your thoughts don't simply reflect your world—they actively shape it. A single negative thought may not define you, but when repeated often enough, it begins to form your beliefs, which in turn influence your actions, habits, and ultimately your reality.

But here's the good news: You have a choice. You don't have to believe everything you think. You can pause, observe, and consciously shift the narrative. Just as you wouldn't let weeds overrun a garden, don't let unhelpful thoughts run wild in your mind. With consistent awareness, you can plant thoughts rooted in peace, resilience, purpose, and self-worth—and watch your life begin to reflect that inner landscape.

Today, be mindful of the stories you tell yourself. When negative thoughts appear, gently challenge them: *Does this story serve my highest good?* Then choose better. Your future grows from the thoughts you plant today, so plant wisely.

What kind of reality do you want your thoughts to create?

TRUE PASSION

True passion is about what you're willing to fight for, endure for, and never give up on.

Passion is often misunderstood. It's not just a spark of enthusiasm or a fleeting moment of excitement. Real passion, the kind that runs deep in your spirit, anchors you in purpose and continues to pull you forward even when the path gets rocky. True passion is what shows up after the initial thrill has faded, after the applause has quieted, after doubt has crept in.

True passion is grit. It's what keeps you going when results have stalled and the road gets long. It's the fuel behind every late night, every quiet sacrifice, every time you choose to try and try again. Passion doesn't just say, "I love this." Passion says, "I'm in this—no matter what."

Passion doesn't just come to you while you sit around waiting. You build passion by staying committed to what makes you feel alive—even when no one else understands.

Ask yourself: *What matters enough that I'm willing to fight for it, even when comfort lures me to quit?* That's where passion lives. Beyond chasing what excites you, fight for what endures.

Where in your life are you being called to show up with more heart, more resilience, and more purpose?

THE DANCE OF RESILIENCE

The strongest people aren't immune to stumbling. But instead of staying down, they stand up and keep going.

Resilience isn't about avoiding the fall. The falls happen no matter how well we plan. True resilience is how gracefully you get up after the fall and take those next steps. Life is unpredictable. Missteps are inevitable. Plans falter. Emotions surge. Challenges knock us off balance. Pretending to be unshakable isn't the answer. Picking yourself up, regrouping, realigning, and reengaging—*that* is the sign of deep perseverance.

The strongest people aren't immune to failure. They've simply made peace with it. They treat each stumble as a cue rather than a condemnation. Each stutter-step backward is a chance to regain their balance. Like a dancer who loses their footing but regains their rhythm, resilient people don't freeze in shame—they flow forward with wisdom.

Each stumble, each fall, each shuffle can become part of the choreography of your life, shaping your grace, your grit, and your growth.

Whenever you fall—emotionally, professionally, personally—pause only long enough to catch your breath. Then stand up, not with self-judgment but with self-compassion. Dust yourself off and let resilience lead. Life isn't about never falling but rather learning how to rise again and again.

What part of your dance is waiting for a graceful return?

DON'T WAIT FOR SOMEDAY

Don't run out of life before you run out of time.

Time moves forward whether we notice or not. But real life requires our presence. Too often, we wait—for better timing, more clarity, fewer distractions. We wait for permission, for certainty, for fear to go away. And while we're waiting, time keeps moving forward. It doesn't pause. Days pass, dreams drift, and we forget that living is more than existing. Yet, living is about being fully awake to the precious moments we're given. It's about laughter, risk, purpose, and love.

Running out of life doesn't equate with running out of time. Running out of life is when you reach the end of depth, of aliveness, of purpose and meaning. And far too often, this happens *long* before the clock stops ticking.

But there's good news: You can choose to live your life fully at any moment, including this one. You have the opportunity to live fully *right now.*

Ask yourself today: *Am I truly living, or am I just getting through the day?* What one thing can you do today to reconnect with life—to feel more, to risk more, to experience more? Life doesn't start later. It's happening right this moment, in every choice you make.

How will you make this moment matter?

OCTOBER 5

CLIMB WITH PURPOSE

Pick your mountains. Not every hill is worth climbing.

You don't need to climb every mountain you see—only the ones that move you closer to who you're meant to become. When you pour energy into scaling peaks never meant for you, you end up too tired to reach the summits that matter.

Many of us have been taught that pushing harder shows how much we care, but effort without direction just leads to exhaustion and burnout. Not every challenge deserves your time. Not every opinion needs a response. Not every task is worth doing.

The real flex? Knowing when to walk away, when to say no, when to channel your power where it truly matters. Growth comes when you move past indiscriminately draining your energy into anything you *can* do and instead choose to invest your energy in action that fuels your higher purpose.

Before you commit your time, ask: *Does this serve my greater purpose? Or is this just another thing to do?* Choose wisely and let go of activities that deplete you. Life will always offer more hills than you can climb. But the mountains that matter—the ones that call your soul higher—deserve your best. Focus your strength where it counts, and your journey will feel lighter, clearer, and far more fulfilling.

What mountains are you climbing today? Are they yours to climb?

SHAPING MINDS

Every word we say, every action we take, molds our children's future.

Children don't just listen. Children absorb. Every move you make, every word that slips out of your mouth, every reaction to disappointment, every interaction with a stranger, becomes part of the blueprint children use to map out their understanding of the world. Even in those moments that seem inconsequential, children are taking notes.

Whether you're a parent, mentor, teacher, or simply in a child's orbit, your influence is profound. You're not just teaching with lessons; you're teaching through presence. The way you handle challenges, offer kindness, manage anger, stand firm in values—all of it leaves an imprint.

In every moment, you are shaping minds and modeling behavior. It's vital to maintain a deep awareness that the next generation is watching and absorbing your every move.

Be intentional with your influence. Speak with purpose, and act with integrity. Recognize that even the smallest moments and interactions can plant powerful seeds in a young mind. Let your words and actions serve as tools that build strength, compassion, and resilience in the little ones who are watching your every move.

What values are you modeling for the next generation, and how can you lead with more intention today?

THE PURPOSE OF SELF-CARE

You can't show up fully for others if you're running on empty.

Many of us have worn exhaustion like a badge of honor, believing that the more we give, the more we matter. But pouring from an empty cup only leads to burnout, resentment, and disconnection.

When we start treating self-care as essential rather than optional, we begin to show up differently. We have more energy, more clarity, more ability to be present. You may think *self-care* sounds indulgent, but it isn't. True self-care is maintenance for your mind, body, and spirit. It's in the strength to say no to yet another commitment when your plate is already full. It's in the courage to step away from your screen, go for a walk in nature, nourish your body with healthy food, or protect your bedtime like it matters—because it does.

The more we take care of ourselves, the more powerfully we can care for those around us over the long haul.

Pause and check in with yourself. Are you tending to your own well-being, or are you constantly placing it last? Make space today for something that nourishes you. Whether it's silence, movement, laughter, or rest, claim it without guilt.

What can you give to yourself today so you can offer your best to the world tomorrow?

SHIFT THE FOCUS

Stop focusing on what someone else did and start choosing how you will move forward.

Every redemption story has a turning point—the moment when the main character stops being defined by what happened and starts choosing what happens next. The narrative shifts when we stop obsessing over the pain, the betrayal, the unfairness, and we reclaim the pen.

Healing doesn't mean forgetting. It means freeing yourself from the grip of what happened and choosing how you will move forward. Yes, it hurt. Yes, it changed you. But it doesn't get to define you unless you let it. When you choose presence over blame and growth over bitterness, something incredible happens: Your power returns. You stop waiting for an apology. You quit needing closure. In walking away from the past, you walk toward something real, something new, something yours.

You will find the beginning of a deeper freedom here—not in the absence of pain, but in the presence of purpose. You become the author, not the aftermath. You rise, not in spite of it, but because of it.

Let go of needing someone else to make it right. Shift your focus. What matters now is *your* next step—and the strength it takes to take it.

What's one decision you can make today that reflects your power, not your pain?

OCTOBER 9

THE FIRST MEETING

To know others, truly and completely,
you must first know yourself.

Learning to understand others often looks like listening, observing, or empathizing. But the deepest form of connection doesn't begin externally but rather within. Many people go through life wearing masks, trying to fit in, protect themselves, or live up to someone else's expectations. But until you're willing to sit with your true self—with honesty and compassion—you'll only ever see fragments of others through the fog of your own unresolved story.

When you have the courage to meet yourself as you are, not as you pretend to be, you will begin to understand others as well—not from a place of projection but from your awareness of your own presence. Meet yourself first, and you will open the door to meeting so many others.

Pause for a moment today and look inward. What parts of yourself have you been avoiding? What truths have you been afraid to face? Drop the mask, even if just for a moment, and allow yourself to be seen—by you. The more clearly you see yourself, the more deeply you'll connect with others.

What truth are you ready to uncover about yourself? How might uncovering it create deeper understanding?

THE GIFT THAT KEEPS GIVING

The greatest gift is life itself, and the most beautiful part of that gift is that it keeps giving.

Life's most valuable gifts don't always come wrapped in celebration or comfort. Sometimes they show up as challenges, quiet moments, or unexpected turns. The key to receiving these gifts well is *presence*.

When you slow down, you begin to see that every day holds a lesson, a connection, a chance to begin again. But when you're rushing, overthinking, or consumed by fear, you close yourself off to what life has to offer. The more open you become—emotionally, spiritually, and mentally—the more you will receive.

Life keeps giving—not just in big moments but through the little, everyday invitations to grow, love, and live fully.

Take a deep breath. Tune into this moment. What is life offering you right now? A moment of clarity? A challenge that could shape you? A gentle reminder to rest? Be willing to receive that gift, even if it's not what you expected. Gratitude turns ordinary moments into extraordinary gifts. The more open you are, the more you'll discover that life is always reaching out—with wisdom, with wonder, and with another chance to begin.

What is life offering you today? Are you open to receiving it?

THE RHYTHM OF LIFE

Life isn't found in the rush of moments, but in the sacred breath that reminds us to truly live.

In our pursuit of goals and the constant pressure to perform, we often forget that life isn't just about movement—it's about meaning. We race from task to task, rarely pausing to breathe, reflect, or feel. Yet in those rare, intentional pauses—in the breath between the task—life is waiting to reveal what truly matters.

The rhythm of life isn't a frantic sprint. It's a dance of effort and ease, action and stillness. When we slow down enough to notice a sunrise, feel the warmth of sunlight on our skin, or be present with someone we love, we realize that fulfillment doesn't live in the rush. It lives in the noticing, in the choice to be here, now, fully alive. Taking a breath isn't weakness; it's wisdom. It helps us recalibrate, savor, and return to what matters with greater clarity and calm.

Breathe deeply and feel the fullness of *now*. Let go of the rush. Reconnect with the rhythm. Life isn't measured by how much you do, but by how deeply you experience what you're doing.

Where will you create more space to breathe today?

THE EMBER BENEATH THE SMOKE

Don't get lost in the smoke. Trace it back to the ember that started it all.

In the midst of conflict, gossip, or even personal doubt, it's easy to get swept up in the smoke—the noise, the reaction, the distortion. But every fire starts with something small. A spark. A truth. An ember. It may be buried, but it's there.

You don't have to believe every rumor or follow every fear. Instead, slow down. Get curious. What's at the root of what you're hearing—or feeling? Sometimes that ember is a misunderstanding. Sometimes it's an unresolved emotion. And sometimes it's a truth that is quietly asking to be acknowledged. The key is not to chase the smoke but to understand the source of the fire. And when you find the source, you'll be able to respond with clarity.

The next time you're caught in the middle of confusion, conflict, or inner noise, pause and look past the drama. Listen for what is beneath the surface. Find the ember. That's where healing, resolution, and truth begin.

What situation in your life feels clouded right now? What truth might be quietly burning underneath?

THE DECISION TO WIN

Winning isn't an outcome but rather a decision you make before you even begin.

Success begins long before the goal is reached. It begins with a decision—a clear and powerful commitment to show up fully, to give your best, and to keep going when comfort tempts you to stop or settle for less.

Winning isn't reserved for the lucky or the naturally gifted; it's claimed by those who choose to pursue it with unwavering intent. That choice fuels your preparation, sharpens your mindset, and anchors your resolve when challenges arise. When you decide to win, even before taking the first step, you align every subsequent action with the outcome you've committed to.

You may stumble along the way, but your decision to win has already been made.

Before you face your next challenge—whether it's a project, a performance, or a personal goal—ask yourself: *Have I decided I am going to win?* You're not just going to try or hope. Decide now. Let that intention shape how you prepare, how you respond, and how you move forward. Because the moment you decide there is no alternative, you've already begun to succeed.

Where in your life have you been "trying," and what would shift if you finally decided to win?

THE POWER OF DOING

The problem and the possible are divided by a single choice: the choice to complain or act.

It's natural to feel overwhelmed, frustrated, or dissatisfied at times. We all have moments when we want to vent, to name what's wrong, to express what feels unfair. But while complaints may feel like release, they rarely lead to resolution. Progress doesn't come from echoing problems—it comes from engaging with solutions.

That doesn't mean you have to have it all figured out. But it does means you need to begin. A single shift, a small decision, an intentional action—that's how change happens. Between what's broken and what's possible lies one powerful moment: the choice to act. And that choice, made again and again, becomes transformation.

While complaining may cause a ruckus, action is louder than noise. It speaks of courage, ownership, and momentum. You don't need to be perfect. You don't need the full plan. You just need to start *doing*.

When frustration about a situation arises, ask yourself: *What's one thing I can do to address this right now?* Then do that thing. It might be small, but it is something. Let your actions move you forward—not just toward an outcome but in pursuit of the strength you build in the process.

Will you use your energy to complain or to create?

THE POWER OF ALIGNMENT

When your values match your actions,
peace becomes your natural state.

A quiet strength arises when you're no longer at war with yourself. Alignment isn't about living a perfect life, never making mistakes or stumbling. Alignment is choosing to live a *true* life—one that acknowledges when mistakes or missteps happen.

When your actions reflect your values, you no longer feel the inner tug of contradiction. You stop second-guessing your worth, your choices, your path. You start living with clarity, intention, and self-respect. It's not always easy. Alignment often requires courage and may mean setting new boundaries, saying no more often, or walking away from things that look good but feel wrong.

But the reward is profound: peace—the kind that echoes within you and reverberates out to others, quelling the need for external permission to feel whole.

Take a deep breath and ask yourself: *Where in my life am I out of sync with what I truly believe? Do my actions match my values?* Realignment doesn't have to be drastic. It can begin with one honest action. Choose one thing today that reflects your values more clearly. Live it. Breathe it. Let it remind you of who you are and what truly matters.

What decision will you make today to move closer to the peace that's waiting within your alignment?

THE WISDOM OF REPETITION

Wisdom isn't only about knowing what needs to change but also what should be repeated.

The world around us moves so quickly and celebrates constant innovation and reinvention. We're often told that progress means leaving the old behind. But true wisdom teaches us otherwise. Sometimes growth does ask us to change direction, but growth also occurs when we recognize the practices, people, and principles that continue to serve us well.

Consistency holds immense value. In fact, some of the most meaningful breakthroughs come not from doing something new, but from doing something meaningful *again*. Wisdom gives us the ability to pause and ask: *Is this helping or hindering me?* If the action uplifts, anchors, or fuels your growth, it deserves to be repeated—not out of habit, but out of honor. This repetition can become a grounding force in a world of distractions.

Today, instead of focusing only on what you should change, take a moment to identify what you should preserve. What habits bring you peace? What actions align with your values? What relationships add depth to your life? These are your foundation—build them up. Wisdom isn't just about evolving but about identifying what's worth maintaining.

What area of your life is quietly working? How can you replicate it with intention?

CREATE SPACE FOR PEACE

Trying to change other people will only drain you. Accepting them will bring peace.

We can't control how others think, feel, or evolve. Maybe we wish someone were more present, more dependable, more open. But trying to force change only leads to exhaustion. Their growth is theirs to own. Acceptance doesn't mean excusing harmful behavior—it means recognizing what's not ours to fix. We can set boundaries. We can express our needs. But we can't rewrite someone else's story, only choose how we show up in our own.

Choosing to accept a person as they are is a sign of deep wisdom. When we meet people where they are and stop carrying the burden of who we think they should be, we create space for peace, our steps become lighter, and we allow others the dignity of their own journey.

Not everyone will match your pace. And that's okay. When you release control and choose understanding over resistance, you protect your peace and honor theirs.

Think of someone you may have been trying to change. *Why* are you trying to change them? What would shift if you simply allowed them to *be*? Practice acceptance today—not as surrender but as an exercise of true strength.

What expectation placed on another person could you release today? How might that create more peace for both of you?

YOU AREN'T WHAT YOU THINK

The voice within can either guide or mislead.
Listen, but then let wisdom take the lead.

That voice in our heads speaks often—constantly, in fact. Sometimes it encourages, sometimes it questions, and sometimes it whispers fear-fueled lies disguised as truth. Here's what you need to remember: Not everything your inner voice says deserves the final word. You are not the sum of your passing thoughts.

Your inner dialogue can be your greatest ally or your sharpest critic. The difference lies in how you listen. When you respond with wisdom—with clarity, compassion, and truth—you reclaim your power. The goal isn't to silence the voice but to listen to and guide it—to allow your highest self, not your loudest fear, to steer your choices.

Thoughts come and go, but your truth remains steady beneath the noise. Learn to recognize and amplify that voice—the voice that's calm rather than chaotic, gentle rather than loud—and let it lead.

When doubt rises, pause and ask: *Is this voice rooted in fear or in growth?* You get to choose which voice speaks the loudest. Let that choice be guided by wisdom rather than worry.

What inner narrative are you ready to rewrite today?

RECLAIMING POWER FROM ANXIETY

When you see anxiety as a visitor—not as your identity—you take back your power.

Many people experience anxiety. And for some of us, it may feel as if it's an inextricable part of who we are—something permanent, unshakable, and inseparable. But anxiety is not your identity. Yes, it's powerful. But it isn't who you are at your core. It's simply an experience, a signal, a visitor.

When we begin to observe our anxiety rather than be controlled by it, we create space to breathe, choose, and respond with intention instead of reaction. That shift doesn't eliminate what we feel inside, but it does loosen anxiety's grip.

Anxiety may knock at the door, but it doesn't get to move in and take over.

The next time anxiety surfaces, notice the language you use around it. Instead of "I am anxious," try "I am experiencing anxiety." That distinction can help shift your perspective and give you space to navigate through the anxious moment. Ground yourself in the present, breathe deeply, and trust your capacity to stay steady. And remember: You are not your anxiety.

How can you begin to observe your anxiety instead of becoming it?

DISCIPLINE IS SELF-LOVE

Discipline is a form of self-love, not punishment.

Discipline is often seen as something rigid, cold, or even punishing—follow this schedule, don't deviate from routine, check off the tasks. But in truth, at its highest form, discipline is a profound act of love.

Discipline means choosing what's best for you, not just what's easy. It's the daily practice of showing up for your well-being, your values, and your future self. That might look like building healthy habits, committing to meditation, or simply getting some sun on your face. True discipline isn't about control; it's about commitment. It's the quiet promise you make to honor your potential and give yourself what you truly need. And it isn't fueled by shame or harshness, but by compassion and care.

When we see discipline as a gift instead of a burden, we begin to experience it as a source of energy rather than exhaustion. Growth is no longer something we force; it becomes a by-product of investing in ourselves.

Reframe the way you see your habits and routines. Let your discipline be an expression of self-respect—a reflection of the love you have for the life you want to live.

How would it feel if you treated discipline as a daily act of self-love rather than as a demand for perfection?

GUARD YOUR DREAMS

Stay focused and keep walking the path that leads to your purpose.

Chasing a dream isn't always about taking giant leaps that land you at the finish line. Working toward a dream requires steady focus and quiet discipline—efforts that often feel incremental and go unnoticed by others.

The world offers endless distractions on this journey—conflicting opinions, the distraction of comfort, self-doubt. Each one can pull us from what truly matters. But every time we reconnect with our *why*, we find our footing again. Purpose may light the path, but focus is what keeps us on it for the entire journey. Distractions aren't always loud. Sometimes they look like good opportunities, but not all good opportunities align with our greater goal. We can even be distracted by small, seemingly inconsequential habits that slowly drain our momentum.

Protecting your dreams means being intentional—not just with what you allow in but with what you choose to release as well. Staying the course isn't always easy, but focus is how dreams are kept alive.

What is silently or stealthily pulling you away from your purpose right now? Identify it. Then commit today to reclaiming your focus. Set boundaries. Say no when you need to. Reignite your vision of what could be.

How will you protect your dreams and stay true to your path today?

MASTER YOUR EGO

Don't give your ego everything it wants.

The ego has a way of showing up uninvited—especially when we're chasing success, craving approval, or reacting to criticism. The ego wants to be right. It wants to be seen. It wants to win. And while our ego isn't the enemy, letting it drive our decisions can lead us down a path of frustration, disconnection, and missed opportunity.

Real power lies in our ability to pause before our ego takes the reins and ask: *Is this pride or purpose driving me?* Oftentimes, the most impactful people aren't the loudest in the room; they're the ones who stay rooted in authenticity even when no one's watching.

You don't need to silence your ego. You just need to guide it. Confidence is powerful. But confidence with humility? That's where you find lasting transformation.

Pay attention to the moments when your ego is in control. Ask yourself: *Is the way I'm behaving about growth or about approval? About truth or about validation?* Choose awareness over reaction and humility over performance. You'll find more clarity, connection, and calm when you do.

What would happen if you guided your ego instead of letting your ego lead you?

THE FREEDOM IN UNCERTAINTY

What feels like fear might actually be freedom, gently inviting you to explore what's next.

We often treat uncertainty like a threat—something we must escape or destroy. But uncertainty isn't emptiness; it's potential. It's the open space between chapters, the moment before transformation, the fertile ground where something new can take root. Yes, it's uncomfortable. Yes, it asks more questions than it gives answers. But it also invites creativity, courage, and clarity that don't surface as readily when everything is certain and scripted.

In reality, what feels like fear is often friction against growth. The part of you that craves control may panic in the middle of uncertainty. But the part of you that is ready to evolve knows that this is where the magic begins.

Let uncertainty be a sign, not of danger but of possibility. In that wide-open unknown, you are no longer bound by who you've been—you're free to become who you're meant to be.

When the unknown feels heavy, breathe into it. Don't rush to fill the space. Ask yourself: *What might be trying to grow in the unknown?* Honor the tension, and trust that whatever comes next will meet you in your becoming.

What opportunity might be hidden within the uncertainty you're resisting?

THE PRICE OF PROGRESS

You'll never reach new ground if you refuse to leave the old behind.

Your comfort zone is a sanctuary of familiar routines and beliefs that you guard fiercely. Stepping outside it can feel like walking into a cold, windy day after leaving your warm bed. You naturally resist that chill, clinging to what's familiar even as it slowly stunts your growth.

Inside each of us, a quiet battle rages between the part that longs to grow and the part that fears change. Out of fear—fear of failure, pain, or the unknown—we often settle for familiar limitations. Not because they serve us, but because they feel safe.

But growth requires risk and discomfort. Like using your muscles in training, you must strain to gain strength. It's in the middle of that discomfort where you'll discover how strong and resilient you can be.

Take a moment to reflect: *What safe harbor am I holding on to simply because it's comfortable?* Perhaps it's a secure job that no longer inspires you or a limiting story you keep telling yourself. Let go of whatever you're clinging to. Dare to step beyond that comfort and into the unknown, the very place where growth and transformation live.

What part of your comfort zone is ready to be expanded so your growth can begin?

NEVER TOO LATE

It's never too late to become the healthiest, strongest, most authentic version of you.

Time doesn't disqualify you—mind-set does. The world may whisper that you're too far gone, too old, too set in your ways. But growth doesn't expire. The body still responds. The heart still heals. The soul still longs for alignment.

Whether you're twenty-five or seventy-five, the journey to your strongest, truest self is still possible, and it starts now. You don't have to undo the past. You just have to honor the present. You can eat better today. Move your body today. Speak your truth today. Breathe deeper, dream bigger, and dare to believe again.

You won't find the healthiest version of you in perfection. You'll find it in the willingness to begin again. And again. Because transformation isn't a destination—it's a commitment to yourself, one decision at a time. Every small act of self-care is a declaration: *I matter.*

Don't wait for the perfect moment. This is it. Reclaim your health. Reclaim your strength. Reclaim your truth. The best version of you isn't in the past. It's in the choices you are making right now.

What's one step you can take today to become who you're meant to be?

MOVEMENT AS MEDICINE

Fitness is the only medicine with
no negative side effects.

Fitness is far more than a routine, a discipline, or a path toward an outward goal. Fitness is a powerful form of self-care. It's a prescription not just for a stronger body but for a clearer mind and a more grounded spirit.

On the days when you feel overwhelmed, a simple walk or a workout can shift everything. Intentional physical movement clears the mental fog, calms your nervous system, and reminds you that you are in control of your health. Unlike quick fixes or temporary relief, fitness offers sustainable transformation. Instead of just addressing symptoms, it gets to the root, strengthening who you are from the inside out.

Every time you move with intention, you're reminded that this is the kind of medicine your body and mind truly need—consistent, empowering, and free of side effects.

Start viewing movement as medicine. Whether you choose to walk, stretch, train, or dance, honor your body with purposeful activity. It doesn't have to be perfect, just consistent. Over time, you'll begin to notice the "side effects" of the medicine of movement: improved energy, greater clarity, deeper confidence, and heightened resilience that strengthens every part of your life.

What dose of movement will you give yourself today for the benefit of your whole being?

OCTOBER 27

MORAL CLARITY

Doing the wrong thing for the right reason is still wrong.

Sometimes we find ourselves at a moral crossroads, tempted to cut corners, tell a white lie, or break a minor rule. It's alarmingly easy to convince ourselves that the end justifies the means. If the end goal is noble and not self-serving, what's the harm in getting there a little more easily?

Yet when we compromise our values, we chip away at the foundation of who we are. Over time, these small chips add up, splintering the core of our values and leading us away from the person we aspire to be.

Moral clarity means understanding that right and wrong aren't measured by results—they're defined by intention and action. Choosing what's right, especially when it's difficult or unpopular, is a quiet form of courage—and every time you do it, you strengthen the foundation of your character.

When you're faced with a choice that pushes up against your integrity, ask: *Will this action reflect who I truly want to be? What could be gained or lost if I took the easy way out?* The path of honesty and honor, even if it's harder, strengthens your self-respect and peace.

When have you been tempted to justify a questionable action? What would it look like to choose integrity instead?

THE TRUTH ABOUT HAPPINESS

There are no substitutes for happiness, only distractions that keep you from it.

Happiness often feels elusive because we've been led to believe we need to search for it outside ourselves. We chase promotions, praise, possessions, and fleeting pleasures, hoping they'll deliver the joy we crave. But while those things may offer temporary satisfaction, they rarely lead to lasting fulfillment.

That's because happiness isn't something you find; it's something you uncover from within. Happiness isn't out there waiting to be achieved, like the next level on a video game. Happiness is within you, waiting to be noticed. When we stop running and start looking inward, we realize that what we've been seeking has likely been quietly present all along—in a moment of stillness, a shared laugh, a deep breath, or the comfort of simply being.

Step back from the noise and reflect on what's already good in your life: *What makes my heart feel light? What brings me peace?* Happiness doesn't come from getting more of something. We feel happiness when we begin to notice what already *is*. Give yourself permission to stop chasing and start appreciating.

What in your life right now—small or significant—holds the happiness you've been seeking elsewhere?

OCTOBER 29

LIVING YOUR LEGACY

Legacy is more than what you leave behind. It's how you live today and shape the world around you.

We often think of *legacy* as something written at the end—a final chapter, a tribute carved in stone. But true legacy begins much earlier. It lives in how you show up each day, how you speak, how you serve, how you stand for what matters. Your legacy is being built in the way you make people feel, the principles you live by, and the small, consistent actions that ripple outward.

Legacy isn't about spotlight moments or grand achievements. It's about being present in the lives you touch each day, intentionally and wholeheartedly. Whether you realize it or not, you're writing your legacy right now. Someone is watching. Someone is learning. Someone is being impacted by the way you choose to live in this moment.

Ask yourself: *What story is my life telling right now?* You don't have to wait until later to leave your mark. Make every moment count. Lead with integrity. Speak with heart. Act with purpose. Your legacy isn't what you leave when you're gone; it's how you live in this present moment.

What part of your legacy will you choose to embody today?

THE VOICE OF LOVE

Love speaks honestly; ego hides behind illusion.

There's a subtle yet powerful difference between the voice of love and the voice of ego. Love is steady, clear, and courageous. It comes to you without disguises. It tells the truth, not to harm but to heal. It chooses connection over control, presence over performance. When we act from love, our words carry warmth, our decisions align with values, and our actions invite harmony.

Ego, however, complicates. It dresses up in false confidence, rehearsed lines, and defensiveness. It seeks to impress, protect, and dominate rather than to connect. Ego whispers illusions that create distance where love longs to build closeness. And it can do all of this while masquerading as love.

The challenge—and the opportunity—is to notice which voice is speaking before we act. When we pause and listen closely, it's easy to tell: Love feels expansive; ego feels tight.

Before you speak, decide, or react, take a breath and ask: *Is this response coming from love or from ego?* If it's coming from ego, soften. If it's coming from love, speak boldly. Let your actions be guided by the desire to grow, heal, and connect.

What might shift if you let love—not ego—have the final word today?

FINDING HAPPINESS BEYOND THE SCREEN

Happiness is found in real-life moments of connection, quiet, and reflection.

We scroll, we like, we comment, but do we feel fulfilled? Social media gives us a highlight reel of other people's lives—often people we don't even know—and in the process, we tend to lose touch with our own life. We compare instead of connecting. We consume instead of creating. We chase validation through screens instead of through presence in the moment.

But true happiness isn't pixelated. It's not measured in likes or followers. Joy is the sunlight warming your face in the morning. A friend listening without distraction. Laughter that isn't recorded. Silence that isn't constantly filled. When you unplug—even briefly—you return to yourself. You start to notice the small joys. The calm. The depth. Life isn't found in the scroll—it's found in the stillness we often avoid.

Set down your phone for a while. Look someone in the eyes. Take a walk without documenting it. Give your attention, not just your reaction. Happiness has been waiting for you to log out and look up.

What's one small, real-world moment that could bring you joy if only you were fully present for it?

NOVEMBER

REFOCUS ON YOU

People often fixate on others to avoid acknowledging their own reality.

It's easy to get caught up in someone else's highlight reel, comparing your path to theirs, your struggles to their success. Social media makes it easier than ever to get lost in a world that has nothing to do with you and overwhelm your mind with if-onlys.

But comparison is a subtle thief. Not only does it steal your joy; it also clouds your vision, blurs your confidence, and distracts you from what is truly yours to build. The more attention you give to what others are doing, the less energy you have for your own growth.

The moment you turn inward—the moment you start showing up for your own goals, your own healing, your own vision—you begin to reclaim your power. You're not competing. You're demonstrating your self-respect by acting in alignment with your purpose.

Are you tracking the lives of others while neglecting your own? If so, it's time to come home to yourself. Reclaim and redirect that energy back to yourself. Your path requires your full presence. Your goals deserve your investment. Refocus on your own progress, and watch your life begin to transform.

What might happen if you gave your life the same amount of attention you've been giving everyone else's?

YOUR TRUEST SELF ENDURES

Beneath shadows of despair, your truest self remains undiminished, patiently waiting for you to believe in it.

When you carry extra weight—physically or emotionally—it can feel like the world sees only the heaviness, not the human. And when depression joins the weight, it tells a cruel lie: This is who you are, and who you'll always be. However, beneath the fatigue, beneath the self-doubt, beneath the pain, you are still there, whole and undiminished.

You may not feel like moving. You may not feel like trying. But even in the stagnation, your truest self is calling. Not for perfection—the relentless pressure to get it all right or to fix everything at once. Not for punishment—the self-criticism that tells you you're behind, broken, or not enough. Just for a breath. A step. A whisper of belief that change is still possible. That you are still worthy. That light can return.

This isn't about the number on the scale. It's about reclaiming the *you* who wants to live not just survive.

Start small. Choose movement over shame, compassion over criticism, a deep breath over defeat. You don't need to be fixed—you need to be uncovered.

What is one loving action you can take today to reconnect with the self that still believes in you?

THE BOUNDARIES OF BEING EVERYTHING

You can't be everything to everyone all the time.

At some point, the desire to help, to please, or to prove yourself becomes overwhelming. The yeses pile up, and suddenly everything feels like an avalanche of overcommitment. In a culture that celebrates constant availability and overextending ourselves, it's easy to fall into the trap of trying to meet everyone's needs. But doing so can make you feel drained, resentful, and disconnected from your own well-being.

Recognizing when you're at capacity is not an admission of weakness. It's a display of wisdom. You are acknowledging that your time and energy are finite and that honoring your own needs will allow you to show up more fully and authentically.

You don't need to be available for every request, every emotion, or every demand. You simply need to be present, honest, and intentional with your energy. True alignment flourishes when you stop trying to do it all and instead commit only to what reflects your deepest values.

Take inventory of your commitments. Where are you stretched too thin? Where might a *no* create space for a more meaningful *yes*? Setting boundaries isn't rejection—it's self-respect.

Where in your life can you create space by choosing presence over pressure and alignment over approval?

SIGNALS, NOT VERDICTS

Your feelings are valid, but they aren't facts. They're signals, not verdicts.

Our emotions can overwhelm us at times. We can feel convinced that because we *feel* unworthy, we *are* unworthy. That because we *feel* hopeless, the situation *is* hopeless.

But emotions, as real and intense as they are, are not facts. They're signals, messengers. They show up to alert us that something inside needs care, attention, or a shift. Feeling those feelings—in their full breadth and depth—isn't a mistake. Where we veer off course is when we believe our feelings are the full truth.

When you pause to acknowledge your present emotions without collapsing into them, you leave space for clarity and wisdom to step in. That's when you begin to respond instead of react. That's when your journey begins to shift—not because the emotions disappear, but because you're choosing who's steering the ship.

When emotions swell—anger, fear, sadness, even joy—pause before taking action. Ask yourself: *What is this feeling trying to teach me?* Create space between feeling and response. Remember, you are not your emotion. You are the awareness beneath it, and you have the power to choose what happens next.

How can you become better at listening to and honoring your emotions without letting them define your reality?

REDEFINING YOUR LIMITS

The only certainty worth having is that your limits are lies your fears told you.

Most of the limitations we believe exist in our lives aren't based in reality but rather in fear. Fear whispers that we're not ready, not worthy, not enough. Fear convinces us to stay safe, to stay small.

But the truth is that limits are often just stories—stories crafted by past pain, old failures, or someone else's opinion. And every time you challenge one of those stories, you prove that fear wrong. The moment you step into discomfort, you grow. The moment you choose courage over certainty, you evolve. What you think is the edge of your limits is often just the beginning. There is no ceiling.

Your greatest potential doesn't live within your current limits—it lives just beyond them. And the only way to find that potential is to stop asking, "Can I?" and to start declaring, "Watch me."

Today, challenge one thing you've convinced yourself you "can't" do. Take the step. Make the call. Send the email. Try the new thing. When you stop negotiating with fear, you start building a new reality.

What so-called limit is actually fear wearing the mask of truth? What might happen if you dared to push past it?

GRATITUDE IN THE *NOW*

Someone somewhere is dreaming of the life you're living. Never take for granted what you once prayed for.

It's human nature to keep reaching for more—to chase the next goal, to reach for the next level, to map out the next version of ourselves. But in that constant pursuit, we often overlook the very blessings we once longed for. The job you have, the relationships you cherish, your health, your peace, your home—these may have been distant dreams not long ago. And yet, when they become familiar, we risk seeing them as ordinary.

Gratitude invites us to adjust our lens, reminding us that joy isn't found in whatever might come next but in recognizing what's right in front of us. When we pause to acknowledge and be grateful for how far we've come, we not only feel more content, but we also build the capacity to receive even more with grace.

Take a moment today to reflect not on what's missing from your life but on all that you have. Look around and notice the answered prayers disguised as the norm. Gratitude will turn the life you're living right at this moment into something sacred.

What part of your life today would your past self be amazed to see? Are you taking the time to truly be grateful for it?

THE POWER OF GRATITUDE

People may forget your words, but they will never forget how your gratitude made them feel.

In the noise of daily life, it's easy to overlook the quiet acts of kindness, the subtle efforts, or the simple presence of others. But gratitude has the power to shift all that. It brings awareness to what truly matters: connection, recognition, and humanity.

Gratitude isn't just a response. It's an intention. A heartfelt "thank you" can remind someone of their worth in a world that rarely pauses to notice them. And when you express gratitude sincerely, you create a moment that has echoes far beyond those few words. Whether someone holds the door open for you, offers some kind of support, or simply shows up, acknowledging them says, "I see you. You matter."

Feelings of gratitude stay with us, softening harsh edges, strengthening relationships, and lighting a path forward—for both the giver and the receiver.

Make someone feel seen today. Choose gratitude over assumptions. Communicate your gratitude for others—not just in passing but with your presence. You have the power to brighten someone's day with a few meaningful words.

Who will you thank today? How might that gesture change their day?

WHAT MAKES A MENTOR

The wisest mentors know that real teaching is about connecting honestly and with heart.

The most powerful mentors and leaders aren't the ones with the most credentials, the loudest voices, or the flashiest presentations. They're the ones who show up *real*, with authenticity and humility. They lead not from a pedestal but from shared experience. They don't pretend to have all the answers. Instead, they invite you into the process with them. They understand that the most effective type of teaching includes both honesty and heart.

Teaching shouldn't ever be about impressing others. True mentoring is about *impact*. You won't be flawless—that's not possible for any of us. But your presence—your *full presence*—can have meaningful and lasting impact. When someone teaches from the heart, with honesty and humility, those they are teaching feel seen. And that connection gives space for transformation to take root.

"Perfection" won't inspire. Your presence will. Whether you're guiding others or still learning yourself, know this: Your honesty may be the inspiration someone else has been waiting for.

Who in your life has taught you the most—not through words but through how they showed up?

THE INVITATION IN THE BREAKDOWN

What may feel like falling apart is often
the beginning of falling into place.

We all have moments when everything feels too heavy—our mind is racing, our emotions overflow, or our body simply says, "Enough." In those moments, it's tempting to label ourselves as broken. But breakdowns aren't the end; they're a threshold. They're the soul's way of telling us that something needs to shift, to heal, to be seen.

Often, the unraveling is where our most honest truths surface. Our pain becomes a teacher. The stillness, a reset. Transformation doesn't always begin with clarity. In many cases, it begins with collapse. What you're experiencing isn't failure—it's friction before you take flight. Growth often whispers through exhaustion, anxiety, or unexpected tears.

Our most difficult moments force us to slow down, reflect, and reconnect with what truly matters: purpose, peace, and inner strength. Every breakdown holds wisdom—if you're willing to listen.

If you're in the middle of a hard moment, pause. Take a breath. Don't fight it. *Feel it.* Ask yourself what's coming up from beneath the noise. You might not be breaking down—you might be breaking *through.*

What is this moment trying to awaken in you that you've been too busy—or too afraid—to face?

THE BEST FOR YOU

There is no "best" this or that, only what works best for you.

We're constantly bombarded with advice from "experts" about what's allegedly the "best" for us: the best way to eat, live, work, exercise, succeed. But "best" isn't a universal standard; it's a personal discovery. What brings one person joy, clarity, or growth may not work for another.

You are the expert on your own life. When you pause to notice what truly feels right—what energizes rather than exhausts, what brings peace instead of pressure—you will begin to create a life that's more mindful, one that actually fits you instead of attempting to squeeze you into someone else's mold.

Fulfillment doesn't come from doing what's trending—it comes from doing what's true. And truth is found when you trust yourself. Sometimes that means saying no when everyone else is saying yes. Sometimes it means choosing rest over hustle, solitude over noise, or a path no one else sees—because it's the one that feels right to *you*.

Let go of comparison. Quiet the external voices. Choose what aligns with your energy, values, and vision—even if it's not the popular choice. Remember that the best path is found within you.

What would your life look like if you stopped chasing the so-called best and started choosing what's best for you?

WHERE EMPATHY MEETS VISION

Great leadership isn't built on completed tasks but on connected hearts.

True leadership goes beyond authority or execution—it lives at the crossroads of empathy and vision. Systems and checklists may create structure, but connection is what builds legacy. Titles may say who's in charge, but people follow who they trust. They follow leaders who listen, uplift, and lead with presence, not pressure.

The greatest leaders aren't successful based only on external metrics. They create a culture of emotional safety, emotional intelligence, and belonging, where voices are heard and potential is ignited. A great leader isn't just measured by what is accomplished but by how people grow because of their influence.

When you lead with heart, people don't just follow commands—they *commit*. And in that commitment, excellence follows.

Reflect on how you lead—whether at work, at home, or in your community. Are you checking boxes or cultivating growth? What kind of energy are you bringing into the room? Let your leadership be grounded in humanity, not hierarchy. Leadership is less about being in charge and more about taking care of those in your charge.

What kind of leader are you becoming? How are those you lead growing because of it?

THE MIRROR OF LOVE

Telling yourself "I love you" is one of the most transformative gifts you can give.

One of the most powerful acts of courage is to face your reflection in the mirror and offer it love—not for what you've accomplished but simply for who you are. Self-love isn't about vanity or perfection; it's about acceptance. When you extend self-love, you are choosing to see yourself fully—the flaws, the fears, the growth, the grace.

We spend too much of our lives waiting for love to come from someone else. But real love—the kind that heals—starts within. When you say "I love you" to yourself, you reclaim your worth. You're declaring you don't need to earn love; you *embody* love. The first time may feel uncomfortable. But even a whisper of those words can break through old patterns of shame and self-doubt.

Over time, these words will become a source of deep strength. The more you affirm your love inwardly, the more freely you show up in the world—grounded, whole, and enough.

Today, take a moment, look into your own eyes, and say, *I love you*. Let the words settle. Allow them to heal. Not because everything is perfect, but because you finally see yourself clearly.

What would change in your life if love started with your own reflection?

NOVEMBER 13

THE MEASURELESS NATURE OF LOVE

There's no "more" or "less" in love, only presence.

Real love isn't a transaction. It doesn't demand proof, keep score, or seek validation. It doesn't compare, compete, or ask to be measured. True love simply *is*—it's in the way we show up, remain steady, and offer ourselves wholeheartedly in the moment. We often ask, *Am I loving you enough?* Or, *Are they loving me the same way I'm loving them?* But love isn't something to calculate—it's something to experience.

The deepest expressions of love are often the quietest: being there when it matters most, holding space in silence, offering truth with tenderness. Real love doesn't perform. It doesn't push or pretend. It just shows up, and its presence says everything our hearts need to hear.

Stop trying to weigh or evaluate love. Instead, practice being fully present with the people who matter. Listen without distraction. Offer kindness without expectation. Be present without needing to prove anything. Love is strongest when we stop measuring it and start living it.

What will you do today to stop measuring your love and bring more presence into it?

THE SPACE BETWEEN

Between your breath and your thoughts
lies the quiet truth of who you are.

You are not your thoughts. You are not your achievements, your fears, or your past. And you are certainly not the story your inner critic repeats. Beneath all that noise, there's a quiet space—a stillness between your breath and your thoughts—that holds the truth of who you are.

That space isn't loud. It doesn't compete for attention. But it's always there, steady and unwavering. In that stillness, you don't need to perform, prove, or perfect anything at all. You simply *are*. And in that being, you are enough.

Real peace lives in remembering yourself, not in fixing yourself or becoming someone else. Commit to finding the space between, the place where you know you can return to your wholeness. It was never lost—it's always been the center of who you are.

Take a moment today to pause. Breathe. Notice the space between thoughts. That's where your true self lives—calm, clear, and worthy just as you are.

When was the last time you felt your own enoughness—and how can you return to it now, even for a moment?

CREATING YOUR OWN CURRENT

Masters of life don't merely go with the flow. They create the currents that carry them forward.

There's value in being able to adapt, in allowing life to unfold without resistance. But there's a big difference between surrender and passivity. While "going with the flow" can offer peace, it can also lead to drifting aimlessly if it's done without intention. True mastery comes not from floating downstream but from choosing where and how to swim.

The people who create change—internally and externally—don't wait for direction. They *become* the direction. They set their intentions, align their actions, and move with purpose, even when the current attempts to push them back. They create momentum, not just for themselves, but for others who are silently waiting to be led by example. Life doesn't just happen to them—*they* happen to *life*.

Take a look at the areas in your life in which you've been coasting. Is it in your work? Your relationships? Your well-being? Instead of waiting for clarity, *create* clarity. Instead of hoping for change, *be* change. Start paddling in the direction of your values. And trust your ability to steer.

What current will you create today, and who might be carried along in it with you?

STAY STEADY

Someone will always try to throw you off course.
Stay steady and keep moving forward.

Distractions and doubt often come from those who can't see the vision you're pursuing. It's easy to let outside voices shake your confidence, especially when you're already navigating your own inner storms. But staying steady, anchored in your purpose, is where your power lives.

Some will misunderstand your path. Others might envy your progress. But their noise doesn't affect your worth, nor should it alter your direction. What matters is how you respond. Will you get pulled off course, or will you stay rooted in your truth?

Our most defining moments often come quietly, through persistence and without any applause. Keep your focus. Protect your energy. Your progress will continue to build as you show up again and again, no matter who's watching or doubting.

The next time someone tries to throw you off track, take a breath. Pause. Reconnect with your *why*. Let your actions speak louder than their opinions. Your journey is yours alone. Honor it with unwavering focus and forward motion.

Where in your life do you need to stay steady despite the noise around you?

THE COMPOUNDING POWER OF PURPOSE

Time spent aligned with your purpose compounds like interest.

The most fulfilling progress doesn't come from scattered effort. Real progress comes from alignment and focus. When your time, energy, and intentions align with what matters most to you, the results go far beyond productivity. They bring clarity, momentum, and meaning. Like compounding interest, every intentional moment builds on the last, quietly but powerfully.

If you've ever felt stuck or overwhelmed, it's likely not due to lack of effort. You may have invested energy in things that didn't truly light you up. When you reconnect with what fuels your spirit, everything begins to shift. Focus sharpens. Motivation returns. Your steps become more deliberate, more effective, freer.

When you move from a place of purpose, not only do you get things done; you also move your life forward in the direction that actually matters.

Reflect on how you're investing your time. Are your daily actions aligned with the person you want to become and the legacy you want to leave? Start small if you must, but do start. And stay consistent. One focused hour today is worth more than ten spent in distraction.

If time is your investment, are you spending it on what truly grows the life you're meant to live?

THE JOURNEY OF PARENTHOOD

Parenthood is the opportunity to journey life's path again, but this time through someone else's eyes.

Guiding another life is full of responsibilities and milestones. But there's far more to this journey than leading. Every time you walk beside a child, a student, a mentee, or reflect on your own childhood, you rediscover pieces of yourself. Their wonder can reawaken your curiosity. Their struggles can remind you of resilience. Their questions can challenge you to reflect more deeply. In a way, you're walking the road again, right alongside them.

If you are the child—whether young or grown—you hold up a mirror for parents or mentors. Your perspective invites them to see the world anew, to soften where they've hardened, to heal where they've been hurt. Your path is uniquely yours, yet it can awaken growth in those who walk beside you.

How humbling and beautiful to realize that in helping another grow, we are also learning, healing, and rediscovering ourselves.

Pause and reflect on the influence you've had—or received—through a shared journey. What have you relearned through another's eyes? What joys have you discovered? What healing have you found? How might you walk with even more compassion, patience, and wonder?

What part of your own life journey has parenthood helped you to walk again—with more meaning this time?

THE SILENT STORM

Long before the first words are exchanged, conflict can begin brewing in unspoken feelings and unresolved tensions.

Conflict rarely arrives unannounced. It often brews quietly—through unmet needs, unspoken fears, and misread intentions. At times, denial of any problem can *feel* like peace because nothing's being challenged on the surface, but in reality, denial is a holding pattern for emotions that are waiting to erupt. It's easy to keep things buried—to stay quiet, avoid discomfort, or maintain the illusion that everything is fine. But beneath the surface, tension is growing. And what starts as a small misalignment can quickly turn into a raging storm.

When you choose to acknowledge and to speak out, with the aim of revealing rather than accusing, you can stop that storm from gaining momentum. You're not creating conflict. You're creating a space where healing can happen.

Peace is found in connection. And connection begins when you give yourself—and others—the chance to be heard, seen, and understood before the storm erupts.

Ask yourself today: *What hasn't been said that needs to be?* Take a breath. Reach out to that person. Start the conversation that could clear the clouds. Your communication doesn't have to be perfect or have total resolution. It just needs to be authentic.

What truth are you ready to speak before the storm arrives?

THE MIRROR OF JOURNALING

A journal isn't merely paper and ink but rather a mirror that never lies.

Many of us have tried to journal over the years, with mixed results. But journaling is more than a positive habit. Journaling is a powerful form of truth-telling. When you sit down to write, you enter a sacred space where masks fall away and thoughts are free to flow safely.

The page doesn't demand perfection. It doesn't judge, interrupt, or reject. It simply reflects. And in that reflection, you can begin to hear your inner voice—one that often gets drowned out in the noise of daily life. Some entries might be messy, scattered, or raw. Some might be mundane. But within all if it lie the seeds of clarity.

Over time, as journaling becomes more comfortable, you'll be less concerned about how eloquently you write and more committed to showing up vulnerably. The page becomes your mirror, reflecting your spirit back to you.

Open a notebook today and spend a few moments writing honestly—no filters, no performance, just your truth. It may feel scary at first, but allow your thoughts to land exactly as they are, trusting that your journal will hold them with grace.

What truth is waiting to be written down today? Are you ready to be brave and face it?

THE SOURCE OF YOUR WORTH

Your worth isn't decided by others. Your worth is a truth you already possess.

Self-worth is so easily misunderstood and so difficult to grab hold of. Many of us spend years chasing approval, hoping that someone else's recognition will finally prove our value. But self-worth doesn't originate outside us. Self-worth begins within. It isn't found in titles, appearances, or praise, and it's not dependent on others noticing or affirming you.

The turning point comes when you stop waiting to be chosen and instead realize that you already belong—to yourself. Owning your worth is less about proving and more about remembering. It's about peeling back the layers of self-doubt until you uncover the unshakable truth: You've been enough all along.

External validation is merely an echo of what you must first declare for yourself: that you are worthy simply because you exist. Don't wait for the echo—be the source.

Pause for a moment and ask: *How am I defining my worth? Am I measuring it based on someone else's words, actions, or attention? Or does my worth rest with me?* Reclaim your worth. Stand tall, breathe deeply, and say to yourself: *I am already enough.* Then let your actions flow from that truth.

How would your life change if you stopped seeking permission to feel worthy and simply believed it?

HOW CAN I SERVE?

"How can I serve?" is a better question to ask instead of "What can I gain?"

Life begins to feel deeper and more meaningful when we stop asking what the world owes us and instead start asking what we can offer it. Many of us start out chasing goals rooted in ambition, achievement, or validation. But fulfillment often comes not from achieving or acquiring but from giving.

Service doesn't have to be grand. Small acts—listening without judgment, showing up for someone, offering kindness without expectation—make a big impact. Your ego may naturally seek praise, but the heart finds joy in presence and connection.

When we shift from chasing rewards to being of service, connection takes competition's place. In that shift, you will feel your purpose rising. Your life will seem fuller. And when we give freely, we often end up receiving more than we gave—more clarity, peace, purpose, fulfillment, and the kind of connection that can't be bought.

Ask yourself today: *How can I serve?* It could be a quiet act of kindness, a moment of patience, or offering your time without expectation. Shift your mind-set from "What do I get?" to "How can I give?" and notice how your heart opens.

Are you living from your ego's grip or from your heart's desire to serve?

THE QUIET CONVERSATION

One of the bravest things you can do is sit still and tell yourself the truth.

Silence can feel uncomfortable, so we fill it with distractions—social media, constant activity, nonstop conversation, overworking, background noise, anything to avoid what we don't want to face. But the most important conversations don't happen outside us. They happen within.

In those quiet moments, when nothing can distract us from a conversation with ourselves, truth begins to surface. The ego may try to rush in with fear, defensiveness, or justification, but when we gently set it aside, we make space for something more honest to emerge—clarity, purpose, insight. Stillness creates space—not just for rest, but for revelation.

Whether you're a young person searching for direction or an adult feeling stuck, silence can be a mirror. It's not always easy to look into it, but often it will reveal exactly what we need to see so we can move forward with intention and truth.

Take five to ten minutes today just for you—no phone, no distractions. Sit quietly, breathe deeply, and ask: *What truth am I ready to hear?* Let the answers flow without judgment. Do this regularly, and you'll notice a shift—more clarity, more courage, more connection to who you really are.

How will you make space to allow your inner truth to be heard today?

THE END OF REACHING

Ego chases more and more—always reaching,
never resting, and never finding peace.

The ego is a restless force. It pushes us to chase success, perfection, praise—to seek more, be more, prove more. Ego thrives on comparison and control, convincing us that fulfillment lives somewhere just beyond where we are. But the more we reach, the more peace drifts just out of our grasp. Because peace doesn't shout. It doesn't chase. It waits quietly in the spaces we've been too busy to notice.

True contentment doesn't come from striving but from surrender. From recognizing that you are already whole. Already worthy. Already enough. And that when you let go, you aren't giving up. You're waking up—maybe for the first time. The end of reaching is the moment you stop performing for the world and return to yourself.

Notice the places where your ego is still in the driver's seat—where it's steering you to prove, to earn, to perform. Then pause and take a few breaths. Commit to choosing stillness over striving and presence over proving. Because peace isn't found in the chase but when you finally let go.

What are you still trying to earn—that you may already be?

NOVEMBER 25

THE TIME IS NOW

If you don't start today, then when?

A moment comes for all of us—a pause, a hesitation—when we consider waiting "just a little longer" before beginning something new. We tell ourselves we need to be more prepared, more confident, more ready. But that moment of delay often becomes a habit, pushing our dreams further out of reach.

Here's the reality: The perfect time rarely comes. And the most powerful shifts actually happen when we stop waiting and start doing—imperfectly but intentionally. Whether the item on your list is a goal, a decision, or a long-overdue change, waiting won't make it easier. Waiting only deepens the rut.

Action, even the smallest action, is what creates clarity, confidence, and momentum. "If not today, then when?" isn't just a question. It's a wake-up call.

If something's been stirring in your gut—a conversation you've been avoiding, a boundary you need to set, a dream that won't stay quiet—don't wait for the fear to vanish. It won't. But courage doesn't need perfect conditions. It needs movement. Send the message. Block the time. Say what you need to say. Nothing changes until you do.

What have you been putting off—and what's one small action you can take today to bring it closer?

TIME IS YOUR FRIEND

The ticking clock is an illusion that turns presence into panic and potential into burnout.

We often treat time as the enemy—something to outrun, control, or master. But in truth, it's not the clock that drains us; it's our perception of time. We rush through our days, cram our schedules to the limit, and mistake motion for meaning, believing that if we just do more, we'll finally feel accomplished.

But speed and output don't equal success. And urgency, when unchecked, quickly becomes exhaustion. Real presence—the kind that makes room for joy, clarity, and growth—requires us to slow down. Time isn't something to fight against or attempt to manage. Time is something to honor and appreciate. The most valuable moments don't live in the future or the past but rather in the moment you're living right now.

When we anchor ourselves in presence, we reclaim our focus, our energy, and our peace. We stop living by the clock and start living by intention.

Pause today. Take a breath. Choose to be present, not just productive. Let your worth be measured not by what you finish but by how fully you show up.

What might change if you stopped racing the clock and instead aligned yourself with what matters most?

BEING UNAPOLOGETICALLY YOU

You don't need universal approval
to be authentically you.

It's tempting to shape yourself to fit the room, to soften your voice so others feel more comfortable. But every time you trade authenticity for approval, you shrink. And the irony is, no matter how much you bend, there will always be someone who doesn't like your shape.

The truth is, you're not for everyone. And that's not a problem. It's proof that you're real. You weren't born to be universally understood. You were born to be deeply aligned. The people meant for your path will resonate with your truth, not your performance. And the ones who don't? Let them go. That is freedom.

When you stop needing everyone to stay, you start standing firmly in who you are. You begin attracting relationships, opportunities, and experiences that mirror your *real* self, not the edited version.

Let go of the need to be everyone's choice. Be *your own* choice. Speak your truth. Show up whole. The right people will find you—and they will stay.

Where are you reshaping yourself to be accepted? What would shift if you allowed yourself to stand tall, unedited, and unapologetically you?

GO WITH THE FLOW

Nothing in life stands still. Flow with change, and it will carry you forward.

Change isn't your enemy. Change is an invitation!

Life isn't meant to stay still, and neither are you. Everything is constantly shifting—seasons, relationships, pursuits, your sense of self. And the more you resist, the harder the process of growth becomes.

But when you stop clinging to what *was* and begin to trust what *is*, you create space for something new. You weren't made to be fixed in one place. Life is a perpetual journey of growth. And that growth doesn't come from control but rather from surrender, from loosening your grip on how you think things *should* be and opening your hand to how they *are*.

The discomfort of change may be challenging, but it is shaping you. With each move, each new current, each new stream, you uncover strength you didn't know you had.

What change have you been resisting? Take a breath. Get curious. Ask yourself: *What's trying to emerge through this shift?* When you begin to flow, life begins to respond.

What part of you is ready to evolve? What old version of yourself are you willing to release to make that happen?

MOVEMENT ISN'T ALWAYS PROGRESS

Focus fuels progress. One task at a time
transforms vision into reality.

One of the most transformative shifts you can make is learning to direct your energy with purpose. In today's hustle culture, where multitasking and productivity are revered, where "hacks" for doing it all flood our inboxes, it's easy to confuse movement with progress. But more activity doesn't always mean more achievement. In fact, when your energy is scattered across too many things, your impact becomes diluted.

Real progress comes from *focus*. When you channel your attention into fewer, more meaningful actions, you will begin to see more noticeable results. Even a small step, when taken with intention, can lead to significant change.

Focus isn't just a productivity technique. Focus is a force multiplier. It turns chaos into clarity and effort into momentum.

Take a moment to assess where you're expending your energy. Are you pulled in ten directions, or are you moving purposefully in one direction? Choose one task, one step, one goal to focus on today (or even just for the next hour). Give whatever that is your full presence. By narrowing your focus, you'll amplify your effectiveness. And with time, that consistent intention will bring noticeable results.

What would change in your life if you stopped spreading yourself thin and started showing up fully, one moment at a time?

GIVE IT AWAY

Life tends to give to those who give
and take from those who take.

Life has a rhythm—a quiet, invisible cadence that governs how energy moves. When we give—our time, our presence, our care—we tap into that rhythm. We become part of something bigger than ourselves.

Our motivation for giving shouldn't be because we're trying to earn favor but because giving freely aligns with a mind-set of universal abundance. The more we offer, without keeping score, the more life responds in kind. We don't always see the impact immediately, and the return might not look how we expected, but the ripples of giving always come back to us with meaning. In contrast, those who only take—who hoard love, praise, or resources—may experience temporary gain but with a silent cost. Life has a way of withdrawing from what isn't shared.

Giving expands us. Taking without giving shrinks the soul. What flows through you also flows *to* you.

Give something freely today—a compliment, a helping hand, your full attention. Notice how you feel in that moment. Giving doesn't take from you. Instead, you become *wealthier* in ways the world doesn't always measure.

Where can you create flow instead of simply accumulating more?

DECEMBER

DECEMBER 1

THE CHANNEL OF PURPOSE

Your intentions carve the riverbed
through which your purpose flows.

Purpose isn't a prize waiting for you at the finish line. Purpose is a current flowing through your life, shaped by the direction you choose each day. Intentions act as the architects of that flow. They determine where your energy goes, what you pursue, and how you respond to both challenges and opportunities.

Without intention, even the strongest desire for purpose can drift into uncertainty. But when your intentions are clear, consistent, and rooted in authenticity, they shape the course of your actions, like a riverbed guiding the water toward something greater. Even during life's detours, a strong intention keeps you aligned. It redirects your energy back toward meaning when distractions try to pull you away.

Over time, the path you've carved becomes deeper, more defined, and more powerful, carrying not only your purpose but your impact.

Take a moment to reflect on what drives you. Are your daily intentions aligned with what matters most? Begin today with clarity and direction. Let choices informed by intention carve the path. Purpose isn't something you chase. It's something you channel, moment by moment.

What intention will shape your flow today?

THE POWER OF RESET

We find clarity and purpose when we dare to pause, breathe, and begin again with fresh intention.

Starting over doesn't mean denying what's come before; it means honoring our life while choosing not to be bound by it. Every experience, every misstep, every moment of pain is part of your story. But it doesn't have to dictate your next chapter.

Like a system reboot, the reset isn't about forgetting—it's about clearing the clutter, removing the static, and realigning with what matters most. Just like a computer can freeze from too many open programs, so can your mind when overwhelmed by competing demands and emotional noise. Hitting reset doesn't erase your memory—it restores your capacity.

You will find wisdom in the pause. You will find courage in your breath. You will find power in the decision to begin again. You're not starting over from scratch. You're starting from experience. Stronger. Wiser. More prepared to rise.

Give yourself permission to reset without shame. Breathe. Realign. Begin again—not because you failed, but because you're ready to live more fully.

Where in your life do you need a reset, and what would happen if you gave yourself full permission to start fresh today?

WHAT FLOWS THROUGH US

Beneath our differences, we share one simple truth: We're all human, connected by what flows through us.

It's easy to get caught up in what separates us—language, appearance, beliefs, borders. And when we do, empathy fades. We hesitate to help a neighbor because their story looks different from ours. Communities fracture. Nations turn fear into policy and misunderstanding into conflict. History shows that every division, big or small, begins with the illusion of *otherness*. But beneath every surface difference, there's something deeper, something universal: our shared humanity. The color of our blood, the beat of our hearts, the longing to love and be loved—these are the truths that connect us all.

When we strip away all the labels and assumptions, what remains is this: We all carry pain, hope, dreams, and stories. And in that shared current, there is profound belonging. Real unity doesn't require sameness—it requires recognition. It asks us to see with compassion, listen with humility, and lead with empathy. Because when we do, everything changes: how we speak, how we serve, and how we see one another.

> Today, choose to look past the surface. Beyond every difference lies something we all carry: the undeniable truth that we belong to each other.

What might shift if you looked at every person as someone already connected to you—through struggle, spirit, and shared humanity?

RESPECT THROUGH UNDERSTANDING

Real strength isn't found in opposition—
it's found in understanding.

Strength is often misunderstood as the ability to stand firm, defend a point, or win an argument based on our conviction. But real strength and wisdom are more nuanced. When we are able to stay grounded in our truth while remaining open to someone else's perspective, we open the door to new levels of respect.

The world is filled with people who think, feel, and believe differently—and that's a good thing! These differences aren't a threat; they're an opportunity. When we choose to listen rather than resist, to understand rather than attack, we invite growth and relationship. Every perspective offers us a valuable glimpse into a different world.

Choosing to respect and understand others doesn't mean we have to agree with their viewpoint. We're simply choosing connection over conflict. In that consistent action, we build bridges where silence or division might have otherwise filled the gap.

Today, notice how you react when someone challenges your viewpoint. Can you pause and listen instead of rushing to defend yourself? Can you stay open without surrendering your values? Make space for understanding, even in disagreement. The more you understand others, the more deeply you will understand yourself.

How will you practice respect through understanding today?

THE CYCLE OF SELF-DESTRUCTION

When life doesn't go according to plan, act with love and compassion, not punishment.

When life isn't going the way we'd hoped, it's easy to turn inward and blame ourselves. Disappointment can quietly morph into self-punishment, showing up as emotional eating, screen addiction, negative self-talk, or other numbing behaviors. Often these habits are more than just bad choices; they're coping mechanisms when we feel powerless or overwhelmed. But they can't effectively address issues.

Recognizing patterns of self-destruction is powerful. It enables us to see these choices not as personal failures but as signals—as calls for self-compassion, not self-criticism. It's a chance to ask what part of ourselves needs tending when we're defaulting to these behaviors.

When you meet your pain with understanding rather than judgment, you break the cycle. You begin to reclaim your sense of peace, choice, and inner strength. You open the door to healing the moment you choose to respond to yourself with kindness.

When life throws you off course, ask: *Am I responding in a way that nurtures me or punishes me?* Choose self-compassion. Channel your emotions into something healing—movement, art, connection. Your value doesn't disappear when things fall apart. That's when self-love matters most.

What healthy habit or support system can you lean on when life doesn't go as planned?

TRUST THE PROCESS

When confusion sets in, remove the noise, let intuition lead, and watch as the impossible begins to fade away.

Uncertainty can feel so overwhelming—nothing seems clear and the pressure to figure it all out only adds to the weight. In those moments, it's tempting to push harder, to try to think faster or force a solution. But clarity doesn't always respond to pressure. Clarity often greets us in the pause—when we breathe, when we let go of the need to control and instead lean in to trust.

Again and again, transformation begins not with force but with surrender. And in that stillness, something powerful emerges: *intuition*. A quiet knowing that doesn't shout but gently guides. When we stop chasing answers and start listening inward, the fog begins to lift. The mind quiets. Our tension softens. And what once felt impossible becomes manageable through presence and trust in our inner wisdom.

If you're feeling overwhelmed, stop trying to control every outcome. Instead, take a deep breath and ask: *What if I go ahead and just trust the process?* Let go of needing all the answers right now. Your inner knowledge is wiser than you think, and it speaks clearest in silence.

What part of your life is asking you to let go of control and trust the process today?

DECEMBER 7

THE CHASE WITHIN

The tiger isn't chasing you. You're chasing the tiger.

It often feels like we're being hunted—like a tiger is at our heels in the form of deadlines, expectations, pressure to succeed, or fear of falling behind. But if we pause long enough to look closely, we might see that the tiger isn't real at all. It's us. We're the ones doing the chasing—pursuing illusions of perfection, validation, or approval.

The stress we feel isn't always from the world pushing us—it's from us pushing ourselves toward things we never stopped to question. This insight changes everything. It allows us to slow down, breathe, and ask: *Is this urgency real or self-imposed?*

When we let go of the chase and get still, clarity emerges. We reconnect with our purpose, move from reaction to intention, and realize that peace has always been waiting within. And when that happens, the tiger simply walks away.

Today, pause and reflect: *Am I running from fear? Am I chasing something that doesn't serve me?* Step out of the cycle of urgency and into the space of awareness. Break free from the imaginary tiger, and align your steps with what truly matters.

What will you stop chasing today so you can finally find peace where you stand?

THE ART OF SURRENDERING

Meditation isn't silence—it's the practice of gently returning to stillness, again and again.

Many believe inner peace means having no unwanted thoughts, or that stillness only arrives when the mind is quiet. But real stillness isn't about silencing the mind—it's about learning to sit with and surrender to it.

The more we resist what shows up in our inner world, the more power it seems to gain. But when we allow our thoughts to pass through without judgment—acknowledging them, then letting them go—we reclaim our calm. Surrendering doesn't mean giving up or losing control. It means choosing not to struggle, determining to meet the moment as it is, and finding peace even in the presence of distraction.

When your mind feels scattered or noisy, don't fight it. Pause. Breathe. Notice your thoughts, then gently guide your awareness back to the present. Let everything in your mind float through, like clouds in the sky, and return to stillness without pressure. Whether during meditation or daily life, the art of surrendering is about making space for peace, not forcing it.

What might happen if you stopped trying to control your thoughts and started observing them with compassion instead?

THE POWER OF "I CAN"

Sometimes the biggest shift
begins with a quiet "I can."

Transformation doesn't always begin with a roar. Sometimes it starts with a whisper—the quiet, steady voice that says, "I can." Other voices may try to drown out the "I can" with doubt, shame, or fear, but that soft, sure voice of self-belief speaks with an honesty and resilience that cannot be denied.

That whispered "I can" is the first crack in the wall of self-doubt you may have built over years of fear, failure, or comparison. And once that crack opens up, possibility begins to flood in. You don't need to have all the answers. You don't need to feel completely ready. All you need is the courage to believe that something different is possible. That you're worthy. That you're capable.

"I can" is more than a phrase—it's ignition. It's the spark that turns belief into motion, and motion into change.

Start with "I can." Whisper it. Write it down. Believe it. Let that conviction rise. Because sometimes your softest voice is the one that sets you free.

What area of your life has been waiting for your quiet "I can"?

THE FUTURE IN YOUR HANDS

The future begins each day with
every choice we make.

The future isn't as mysterious as the world makes it seem. It's shaped in the quiet, everyday moments presented to each of us—our habits, our mind-set, our decisions.

Every thought you entertain and every action you take adds a brick to the path ahead. From how you treat your body to how you speak to yourself, you're constantly writing tomorrow's story today. You may not control everything that happens, but you do control how you show up.

Your future isn't waiting for some grand breakthrough. Your future is waiting for your consistency. Small choices made with intention become the patterns that shape your destiny. You don't have to see the full map to begin; you just have to take the next right step, again and again.

Every choice you make either builds your future or delays it. If today's steps aren't leading you where you want to go, don't be afraid to pivot. Even one step in the right direction can change everything.

What small action can you take today to make your future self proud?

THE WEIGHT OF EXPECTATIONS

When self-blame rises, it's often not rooted in truth but in an attachment to your expectations.

Sometimes disappointment feels more like failure. When life doesn't unfold the way we'd hoped, we quietly turn the blame inward—not because we've done something wrong, but because reality isn't matching our expectations. But self-blame doesn't usually come from truth. Truth is the acceptance of what actually is—simple, grounding, free of judgment.

Expectations, on the other hand, are heavy and unforgiving. They whisper that you should have done more, been better, or controlled the uncontrollable. You plan the perfect launch, pour in your energy, strive to make it a success—and when it doesn't land the way you hoped, you assume you failed. But maybe it wasn't failure. Maybe it just wasn't meant for now.

Learning to recognize the difference between truth and expectation helps you release shame, gain clarity, and move forward with greater compassion for yourself.

When self-blame begins to creep in, pause and ask: *Am I responding to truth, or am I reacting to an unmet expectation?* Let go of what you thought would happen and make space for what *is*. Growth happens not when everything goes as planned, but when you learn to rise from what didn't.

What expectation do you need to release so you can reclaim your peace?

THE GIFT OF HELPING

Those who help are always helped.
When we lift others, we rise too.

Helping others is one of the most powerful ways we grow. Whether it's offering support to someone in need, encouraging a friend, or simply being present for another person, each act of service invites something deeper to awaken within us.

A quiet strength emerges when we step outside ourselves to uplift someone else. We're able to connect with the best parts of who we are. Our compassion expands. Our gratitude deepens. And often, the light we give away returns to us, guiding us through our own challenges with greater clarity.

Helping others isn't just a kind act; it's a reflection of our highest self. When we help someone else, we're reminded that growth isn't only about what we achieve but about how we show up for one another along the way.

Offer kindness, support, or simply your presence to someone who might need it. Don't underestimate the impact of even the smallest gesture—it could shift someone's entire day. And while you're doing this without expecting anything in return, take a moment to notice how your own spirit rises in the process. Helping is a gift that wraps itself around both the giver and the receiver.

How will you let your light brighten someone's life today?

UNSTOPPABLE MOMENTUM

Your momentum is unstoppable. Every challenge has shaped you. Every step has strengthened you.

You've earned your momentum—not through ease but through effort. Every detour, every delay, every doubt you've stared down has carved a path of resilience beneath your feet.

You didn't wait for perfect conditions. You got started and kept moving. And now a force is at your back that doesn't just push; it propels you forward. Your success isn't luck. It's the result of persistence. Of getting back up when most would have stayed down. Of believing, even when evidence was scarce.

Momentum isn't magic. Momentum is muscle—built up by showing up day after day, even when the finish line isn't visible. And now that you've found your rhythm, don't slow down. Lean into it. You've got more in you, and the best is still unfolding.

Take a moment to honor how far you've come. Let your scars remind you of your strength and your strides remind you what's possible. The path ahead isn't a question—it's an invitation.

What would happen if you stopped doubting your power and started trusting the unstoppable momentum you've already built?

THE WISDOM OF PATIENCE

Patience whispers, "Wait"—not as a pause, but as a promise of what's to come.

Patience isn't passive—it's a form of active trust. It's not about doing nothing; it's about doing the right things even when results can't be seen. In a world wired for instant gratification, patience is a quiet rebellion. Patience asks you to breathe, to believe, and to build without rushing the outcome.

You may not see the full picture yet, but that doesn't mean it isn't forming. Like seeds beneath the soil, growth happens in the dark. What you water with consistency and care will eventually break through. Waiting with wisdom gives you time to prepare. You're not pausing your life; you're working on your alignment in anticipation of what's to come.

When frustration rises, remind yourself: *The delay is not denial.* The space between desire and fulfillment is where character is shaped, strength is tested, and clarity is born.

Instead of resisting the wait, lean into it. Trust the pace of your journey. Stay ready, remain focused, and let patience carry the promise forward.

What if this season of waiting is preparing you for more than you could possibly imagine?

THE LENS OF PERCEPTION

You don't see the world as it is. You see it through the lens of who you are.

We don't just observe the world. We interpret it. Every belief, every past experience, every pattern, and every emotion colors what we see. That's why two people can face the same situation and walk away with completely different experiences and truths.

The lens you look through—crafted by your story—shapes your reality. When you're feeling stuck or discouraged, take a moment to ask: *Is this the world speaking? Or is my lens distorting reality?* If you carry fear, the world feels threatening. If you lead with curiosity, life becomes full of possibility. You have the power to clean the lens—to shift perspective, challenge old narratives, and choose a new view.

You can't always change what happens around you. But you can always adjust how you see it. And sometimes, that shift is the beginning of everything.

Notice the image you're bringing into focus for yourself today. Is it helping you grow or keeping you small? Try shifting the lens. How does the picture change?

What belief or assumption might be coloring how you see your life? Are you willing to look at it differently?

THE ROLE OF REGRET

Regret's purpose is to turn past mistakes into wisdom, not to shape your future.

Regret is a natural part of human experience. We make mistakes; we miss opportunities; we say things we wish we could take back. Sometimes we cause real harm to others and ourselves. But living in a perpetual state of shame doesn't heal wounds or offer forgiveness, and even the biggest mistakes don't separate us from redemption.

Rather than dwelling in regret, we can choose to learn from it. When we allow regret to become a permanent lens, our view of who we are becomes distorted. But when we take it as a moment of reflection and choose to grow and do better, we are accepting an invitation to extract meaning from the past without dragging it into our future.

We all make mistakes. Growth wants us to ask: *What did I miss? What can I do differently the next time? What choice aligns with my values?* In that moment, regret can transform from a chain to a compass.

When regret whispers, listen. But don't engage in an extended conversation. Ask yourself: *What truth is this feeling pointing to? What wisdom is trying to surface?* Thank the lesson, release the shame, and move forward with intention.

What regret are you carrying? How can you shift that regret from guilt to guidance?

SHOW UP TODAY

When you give your all and release the outcome, you've already won—because you showed up fully.

We're often taught to measure success by results—grades, titles, achievements, recognition. However, real fulfillment isn't found in outcomes but rather in the process. Our effort, our intention, the courage it takes to keep showing up, especially when no one is watching, shapes us far more than any so-called success.

When we release the need to control or predict the result, we make space for something deeper and infinitely more rewarding—*presence*. True power and success are built in those moments when we give our full effort without the guarantee of reward.

When you detach from the pressure of outcomes, you will begin to move with more purpose and less fear. Your intentions will become clear. And your confidence will grow—not from the win but from your willingness to commit and to trust yourself in the moment.

Ask yourself: *How am I showing up today?* Give your energy to what you can control—your attitude, your effort, your presence. Let go of the rest. When you stop needing future outcomes to validate your worth, you will begin to fully own your present.

How might your life change if you stopped chasing outcomes and started showing up simply because you believe in what you're doing?

THE WEIGHT OF UNRESOLVED WORRIES

What troubles you by day will torment you by night—
unless you confront it with reason and clarity.

Unspoken worries don't simply vanish. In fact, they seem to multiply in the quiet. What begins as a passing thought can spiral into sleepless nights. During the day, distractions may keep your mind occupied, but at night, as the world grows quiet, silence has a way of amplifying everything you've been avoiding.

And yet most of what keeps us tossing and turning loses its intensity when it's brought into the light of reason. Avoidance may provide temporary relief, but it comes at a steep cost. And the longer we keep that worry in the dark, the bigger it grows.

When you confront your worries with intention, honesty, and self-compassion, you reclaim control. You don't need to have answers. Simply naming your worry, questioning its truth, and addressing what is in your control can shift everything.

Before you go to sleep tonight, pause and check in with your thoughts: *What am I carrying that doesn't need to follow me into tomorrow?* Write it down. Talk it through with someone if you can. Reflect without judgment. Confront your worry, not to fight it but to understand it. And then allow yourself to rest.

What will you face today so you can finally rest tonight?

THE GIFT OF CONSTRUCTIVE CRITICISM

Learning how to give and receive constructive criticism can bring clarity and synergy.

There's a meaningful distinction between being criticized and being guided. Constructive criticism—when offered with care, clarity, and empathy—can become a powerful catalyst for growth. Rather than stinging or being harsh, transformative feedback resonates because it's honest, intentional, and rooted in respect. When the intent is to help rather than harm, criticism evolves into clarity.

In personal relationships, creative work, or professional development, being open to thoughtful feedback will refine your path and strengthen your impact. At the same time, learning to give feedback with kindness and intention helps others grow without fear. It fosters progress and connection—for both parties.

Constructive criticism, when given and received well, becomes a gift. Like when a colleague says, "This message is strong—if you tighten the ending, it'll leave a deeper mark." That's not a dismissal. That's a gift. A mirror handed to you—not to judge, but to sharpen.

The next time you're faced with feedback, receive it as an opportunity. Ask yourself: *What can I learn here?* And be introspective when giving feedback: *Am I trying to help this person grow, or am I simply pointing out flaws?*

How can you use thoughtful criticism to support growth—in yourself and in those around you?

MOVE BEYOND COMFORT

Growth lies beyond your comfort zone,
where reality stretches into possibility.

Comfort may feel safe, but it rarely leads to transformation. The truth is, everything you're capable of—every dream, every breakthrough, every success—lives just beyond what's familiar. Growth doesn't happen in the predictable. It happens in the stretch, in the risk, in the choice to move through discomfort with courage.

You weren't born to stay small. You were born to rise—to evolve, to expand, to become. But to do that, you must be willing to step beyond the familiar. The unknown isn't your enemy—it's your invitation. Every time you choose challenge over ease, uncertainty over routine, you unlock new levels of strength, clarity, and possibility. Don't let your comfort zone become a cage disguised as peace that holds you back from who you're meant to be.

Identify one area in your life where you've played it safe. Why have you done that? What has kept you stuck there? Take one bold step forward. Embrace the stretch. Welcome the discomfort. It means you're growing.

What opportunity might open up if you were to step outside your comfort zone?

UNRAVELING SELF-DESTRUCTION

We often hold on to self-destructive behaviors because we believe they serve us in some way.

It sounds paradoxical. Why would we cling to the very behaviors that harm us? But beneath every self-destructive habit is a hidden reward: Overeating may bring comfort. Avoidance may offer protection. Overworking may disguise a feeling of unworthiness as achievement.

These patterns survive not because we're broken but because, at some point, they helped us cope. However, what once soothed us may now be sabotaging us. And until we recognize the *payoff*, we'll struggle to let go. Change requires honesty, not just about what's hurting us but about *why* we keep inviting it in.

When looking at a behavior you'd like to change, the question isn't: *Why can't I stop?* It's: *What am I getting from this?* Only by meeting the need *behind* the behavior can you replace it with something better. You don't need to punish yourself into change. You just need to understand yourself into healing.

Reflect on a behavior or habit that you know is holding you back. Ask yourself: *What does this behavior give me? What else could meet that need in a healthier way?* Growth begins when you stop judging your patterns and start listening to them.

What "bad habit" might actually be a misunderstood form of protection?

NO QUICK FIXES

If you're searching for a way to get in shape, know that only consistency and effort will get you there.

Getting in shape isn't about shortcuts. It's not about magic diets, secret routines, or hacks that promise transformation with minimal effort.

The often-overlooked truth is simple: Consistency will always beat intensity. Consistent effort over time is what shapes the body, sharpens the mind, and strengthens the spirit. And this effort doesn't have to be perfect. The only requirement is that you keep showing up. There will be days when you feel unmotivated, when progress feels invisible. But remember that every drop of sweat, every repetition, every healthy choice, every step forward is a deposit in the account of long-term success.

Fitness isn't a sprint. It's a decision you commit and recommit to day after day. And the reward goes far beyond appearance. How you *feel*, how you *move*, and how you *live* will tell the story of choosing the right way to get to health.

Stop chasing "easy." Instead, choose real. Choose effort. Choose commitment. The version of you that you're becoming? It's built in the quiet—when no one else is watching, but you show up anyway.

What small action can you commit to today that your future self will thank you for?

RETURNING TO JOY

Happiness is your natural state. If you're unhappy, you've lost sight of it.

We come into this world untouched by comparison, self-doubt, or fear. Joy is our baseline—an inner light that shines not because of what we achieve but because of who we are in the depths of our spirit. But as our lives unfold, we take on layers. Expectations tighten. The noise of the world grows louder than the whisper of our truth. And slowly, we drift from our center.

Unhappiness isn't failure; it's feedback. It's your soul quietly nudging you, reminding you that you've moved too far from center, away from what grounds you. Joy doesn't need to be manufactured, acquired, or chased. It simply needs to be remembered.

Beneath the clutter, beyond the distractions, your happiness is still there—steady, waiting, and whole. Joy won't shout for your attention. It simply waits for your permission to rise again.

When life feels heavy, don't reach outward. Return inward. Strip away the noise. Close your eyes. Ask yourself: *What have I added to this equation that never belonged in the first place?* Then breathe. Release. Reconnect. Joy is waiting to be uncovered.

What could you let go of today to return to the happiness that's always lived within you?

THE SOURCE OF KINDNESS

Kindness begins within. And the more kindness you give yourself, the more you have to give to the world.

Kindness isn't only something we give to others. Kindness is something we must offer ourselves first. Many of us are taught that self-care is selfish, that service should come before rest. But we can't pour from an empty cup. When we neglect our own needs—pushing through exhaustion, ignoring rest, or speaking harshly to ourselves—our ability to be kind to others wanes. It starts to feel forced, and it can even cause us to feel worse about ourselves.

When we choose to pause and look at the person in the mirror, to forgive ourselves and speak gently, everything shifts. We settle into peace. We find more energy, more empathy, and a deeper well of compassion to draw from. Self-kindness isn't indulgent—it's essential. It's the groundwork for genuine connection and sustainable care. The way we treat ourselves sets the tone for how we treat the world.

What act of kindness can you offer yourself today? Maybe it's letting go of guilt, taking a mindful pause, or saying no to something that drains you. Start there. When you treat yourself with care and respect, kindness becomes your natural state and radiates effortlessly to those around you.

How might your relationships shift if you began by being kind to yourself first?

LOVE AND FREEDOM

Love thrives in freedom, not in control.

Love, at its core, is not about holding on tight—it's about letting go with grace. When we try to control someone out of fear, we suffocate the very connection we seek to protect. Possessiveness often disguises itself as care, but beneath it lies insecurity.

True love, on the other hand, offers space. It trusts. It respects. It says, "You are free, and I still choose you." Some of the most meaningful connections don't grow under pressure but in freedom. The moment we stop trying to grip so tightly is the moment we begin to build something real—something that's chosen, not forced.

Examine your relationships, whether romantic, platonic, or familial. Are they rooted in freedom or control? Are you clinging out of fear, or are you showing up with trust? Today, practice loving without the need to possess. Release expectations and focus on presence. Love isn't about keeping someone—it's about choosing them again and again without force.

Where can you shift from fear to freedom in how you give—or receive—love?

THE ILLUSION OF ESCAPE

What you avoid when you escape doesn't vanish; real peace begins where avoidance ends.

Escape may offer a break, but it isn't a way out. When the noise fades, what we've been avoiding is still there—quietly waiting and possibly more urgent. It's natural to want relief—to disconnect, distract, or numb when life feels heavy. We tell ourselves we just need a break, a breather, a way to silence the noise.

The truth is, most forms of escape are only temporary. They offer a pause but no real peace. Because when the distraction fades, the ache remains. The questions return. What you avoid doesn't disappear. It waits—quietly, patiently. And often, it's not there to punish you but to teach you.

Real healing begins when you stop running and start listening. When you face what hurts not with resistance, but with compassion. Avoidance keeps you stuck in cycles. Presence sets you free.

The next time you feel the pull to escape, instead of running, pause and ask: *What am I trying not to feel? What's calling for my attention beneath the urge to check out?* You don't need to solve everything at once. You just need to face it—gently, honestly, one breath at a time.

What might shift in your life if instead of escaping discomfort, you chose to meet it with grace?

STOP RUNNING

True transformation begins when you stop running and start reflecting.

It's easy to believe that a new job, city, or relationship will finally bring the peace you crave. And while fresh starts can offer space to grow, they don't give you the power to outrun what lives inside you. If you keep finding yourself in the same emotional patterns, the problem may not be the place. It may be the pain you're carrying with you.

Sometimes, changing your environment is necessary, but real transformation doesn't come from swapping scenery. It begins when you sit still long enough to face what you've been avoiding. When you stop chasing external change and start doing the inner work, clarity and peace rise to the surface. That's when you uncover the unmet needs, the lingering wounds, and the unspoken truths that have quietly shaped your path.

Healing happens not in escape but in turning inward.

If you're constantly seeking change, pause and look within. Before you move again, ask yourself: *What inside me needs attention rather than distraction?* The peace you seek isn't out there waiting to be found. Peace will grow when you return to yourself.

What discomfort keeps following you? What might it be trying to teach you?

THE STRENGTH TO MOVE FORWARD

When being nice isn't enough, it's time to move on.

Kindness should never cost you your peace. You might find yourself pouring energy into relationships, work, or situations that no longer nourish you—staying hopeful and patient, believing that more effort will eventually make it better.

Maybe it's being constantly available to a friend who only calls when they need something. Or staying in a toxic job because you feel guilty leaving a coworker behind. Or holding on to a relationship that keeps taking without ever giving back. But kindness without boundaries becomes self-betrayal. And being nice is not the same as being whole.

Sometimes, the bravest move is to walk away with grace. Leaving what drains you doesn't make you weak or unkind. It means you're choosing growth over stagnation, self-respect over self-sacrifice, and peace over pleasing. You're not quitting—you're realigning. And that's strength.

If you've given your best—if you've shown up with compassion, honesty, and clarity—and it still isn't enough, give yourself permission to let go. The quiet decision to honor your well-being and move toward a life where you're seen, supported, and empowered is not weakness. It's courage.

Where in your life is it time to stop being nice and start being brave?

THE POWER OF SHIFTING PERSPECTIVE

Perhaps the situation doesn't need to change,
but the way you're looking at it does.

It's easy to get trapped in your own experience, to believe that your struggle is uniquely heavy. But when you pause, step back, and widen your view, your vision may open up. You begin to see that *everyone* is carrying something—sometimes visible, often hidden. That recognition allows empathy to awaken. You realize that the world isn't divided between the strong and the struggling—we are all both.

But it goes deeper. The same perspective that helps you see others more clearly can also set you free. What if the wall in the middle of your path isn't solid but just appears that way from your current angle? What if the obstacle is actually an invitation to reframe?

True growth rarely begins with doing more but instead with seeing your situation differently. Your greatest breakthrough might be hiding in plain sight, waiting for you to question a long-held belief or let go of a narrow view. When you choose to look through a wider lens, life offers new meaning, new solutions, and new strength.

> Today, don't just look at your challenges—look *through* them. Ask: *What else could this mean? What might someone else be carrying?*

What perspective shift could create the breakthrough you've been waiting for?

OWNING YOUR FIGHT

Power begins when you stop waiting to be saved and start owning your fight.

There comes a time when we realize it's time to stop looking outside ourselves for rescue, when we need to stop allowing fear to keep us from acting. Instead, we must pick up the pen and begin writing our own comeback story.

You don't magically step into your power when someone finally sees your pain. Power shows up when *you* show up—when you look yourself in the mirror, drop the excuses, and choose to step into the ring. Self-pity can feel safe, but it's a cage disguised as comfort. Staying stuck in fear or self-pity delays healing, progress, and evolution. True growth happens the moment you stop asking for someone else to fix what you were born capable of transforming.

Choosing to stand tall doesn't mean you're no longer afraid. It means you've decided that your conviction is bigger than your fear. It means you've accepted the challenge to rise up—not despite your struggle but *because* of it.

Don't wait for permission or praise. Don't wait for someone to hand you the courage you already possess. Take a breath, take a step forward, and own the battle that's calling you forward.

Have you been waiting to be rescued? What would shift if you owned your fight instead?

THE LIGHT OF PRESENCE

Fear may cloud the path, but presence sheds new light.

Fear rarely lives in the *now*. Fear feeds on the past (what could have been) and the future (what might go wrong). But the present moment? Peace owns the present. The present, and the peace that comes with it, is where you'll find your power. When your mind races with doubt, pressure, or uncertainty, it's easy to feel lost. But the moment you pause, breathe, and return to the here and now, something shifts.

Stillness creates space. Space invites clarity. And within that clarity, creativity, resilience, and intuition begin to rise. Presence doesn't demand perfection; it simply invites awareness. It doesn't deny fear, but it stops letting fear lead.

The light you're looking for isn't far off in the distance—it's right here in the now. You just have to be still long enough to notice.

If your thoughts are spiraling and fear is speaking loudly, stop and return to your breath, to this moment. Choose presence—not as an escape but as a guide. In presence is strength, wisdom, and, most of all, peace.

Will you give yourself permission to pause and look for your light? What might that look like?

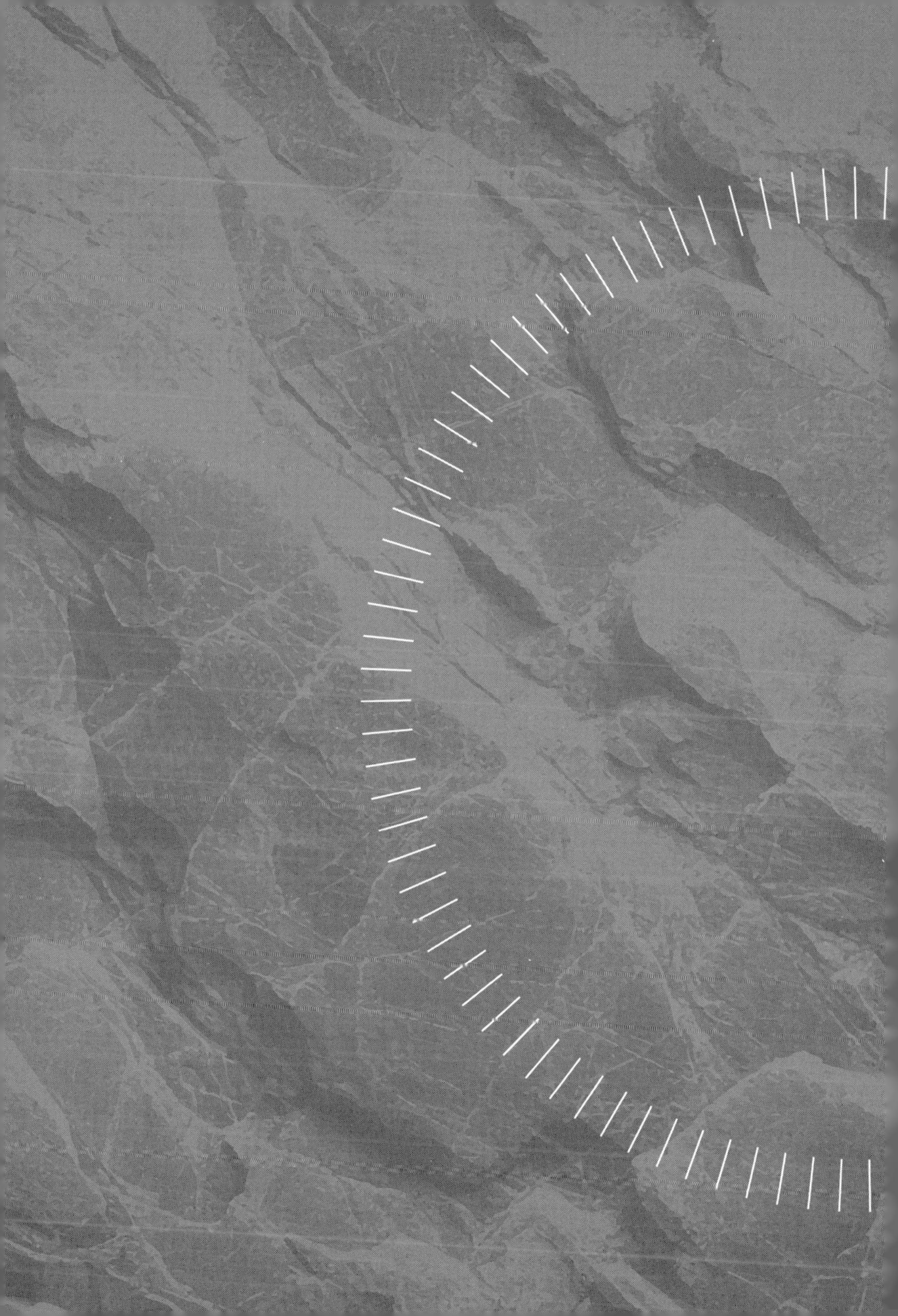

ACKNOWLEDGMENTS

And I did not rise alone.

My strength is stitched from the love and sacrifice of those closest to me. My mother and father—two warriors in their own right—gave everything they had so I could dream beyond borders. My nine sisters and three brothers carried me through the beautiful chaos of a large family, teaching me resilience, loyalty, and the unspoken language of belonging. The women I married and the children I was blessed to bring into this world became both anchor and compass, shaping me in ways that words can never fully capture. If I have become anything worth admiring, it is because of them.

And then there was King. My beloved French bulldog, my healer with four paws and a boundless heart. In his eyes lived a love so steady it could silence storms, a presence so pure it reminded me daily of what truly matters. He was not just

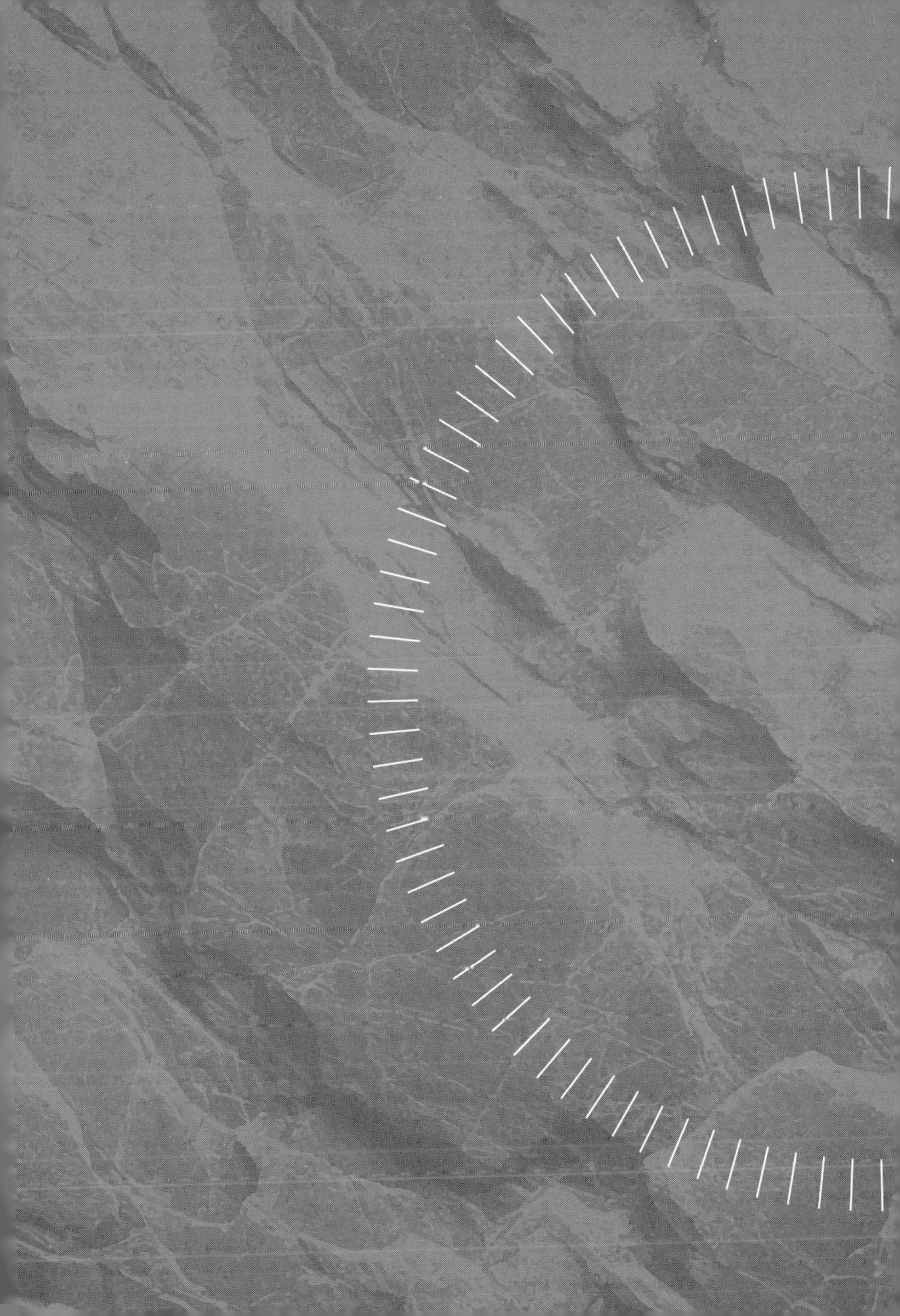

ACKNOWLEDGMENTS

And I did not rise alone.

My strength is stitched from the love and sacrifice of those closest to me. My mother and father—two warriors in their own right—gave everything they had so I could dream beyond borders. My nine sisters and three brothers carried me through the beautiful chaos of a large family, teaching me resilience, loyalty, and the unspoken language of belonging. The women I married and the children I was blessed to bring into this world became both anchor and compass, shaping me in ways that words can never fully capture. If I have become anything worth admiring, it is because of them.

And then there was King. My beloved French bulldog, my healer with four paws and a boundless heart. In his eyes lived a love so steady it could silence storms, a presence so pure it reminded me daily of what truly matters. He was not just my companion—he was my teacher, my mirror, my constant reminder that strength can be soft and that unconditional love is the greatest power of all. His spirit lingers between these pages, and in every lesson I share, there is a trace of him.

To my acquisitions editor, Danielle Peterson, and my publisher, Michael Aulisio—two incredible beings, true dog lovers, and my advocates at Harper Celebrate—thank you for believing in me and for sharing my vision with such heart. To the amazing editors, Alli and Jennifer, whose insight, care, and brilliance elevated every page. To my agent, Cole Lanahan, whose faith in this project never wavered. And to a very special person, who chooses to remain unnamed, but whose trust, love, and generosity of heart carried me further than words can ever acknowledge.

To my family, my friends, my mentors, my clients, and to King—this book is not mine alone. It is ours.

ABOUT THE AUTHOR

Nordine Zouareg is an internationally renowned fitness expert, wellness professional, and anti-bullying advocate. Nordine has claimed titles such as Mr. Europe, Mr. World, and Mr. Universe and has since become a sought-after motivational speaker, high-performance coach, and three-time author whose work has positively impacted thousands worldwide.

Former fitness and wellness director at Miraval Resorts and Spas, Nordine brings a wealth of experience in guiding individuals toward their physical, mental, emotional, and spiritual goals through his uniquely intuitive coaching approach. His holistic wellness program effectively provides the essential energy, guidance, and support to both individuals and groups as they work to overcome obstacles in their lives. He also shares his message of resilience and empowerment as the host of the *No-Limits Life* podcast and through his work with iHeart Radio, reaching global audiences with conversations that inspire real transformation.

Nordine has successfully guided individuals from various backgrounds, including celebrities, CEOs, politicians, athletes, and entrepreneurs, to reach their full potential. Born in the Sahara Desert and raised in France, Nordine now resides in Tucson, Arizona, where he enjoys the desert's stillness and going on hikes.

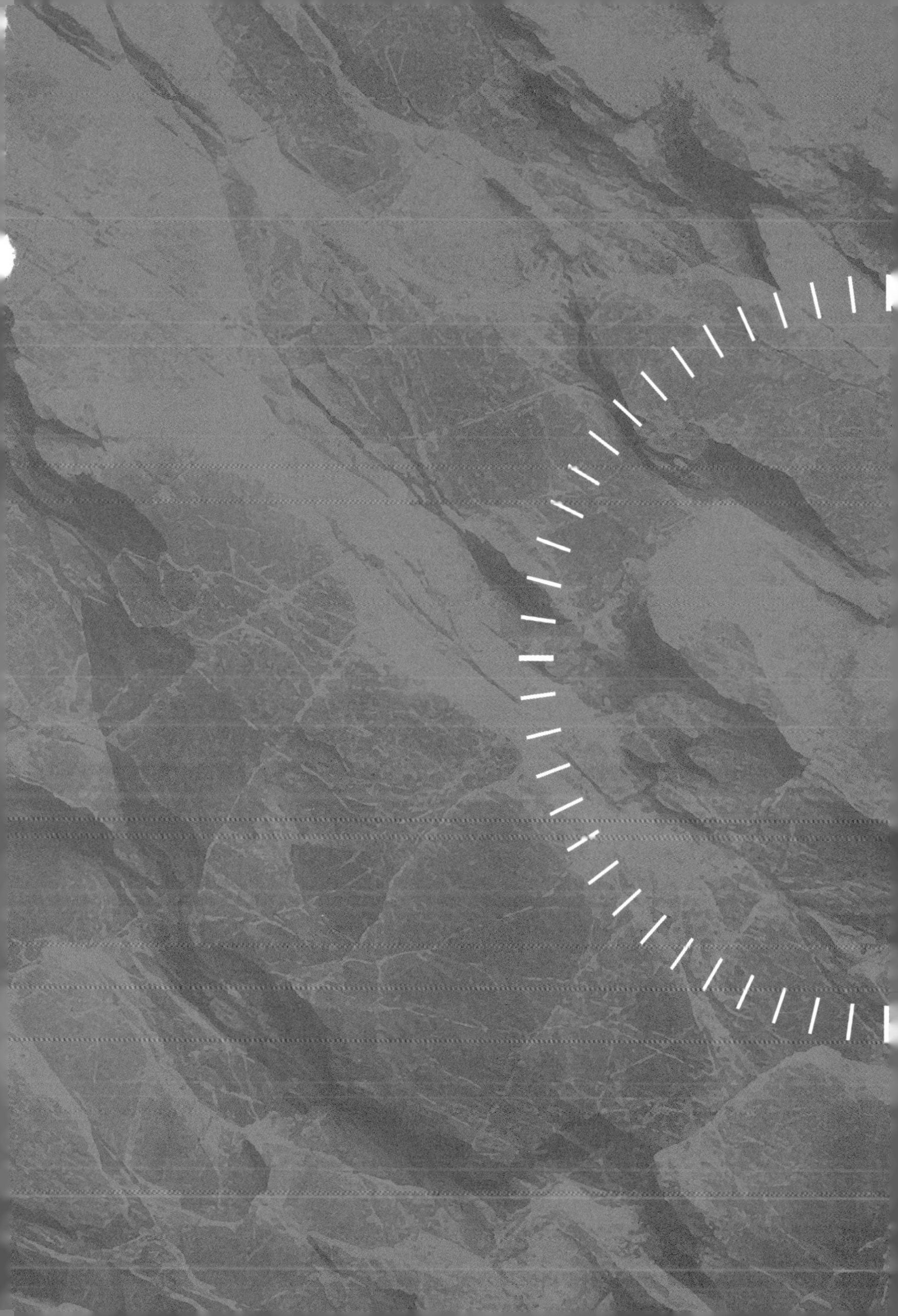